Place and Identity

The UK is experiencing a housing crisis unlike any other. Homelessness is on the increase and more people are at the mercy of landlords due to unaffordable housing. *Place and Identity: The Performance of Home* highlights that the meaning of home is not just found within the bricks and mortar; it is constructed from the network of place, space and identity and the negotiation of conflict between those – it is not a fixed space but a link with land, ancestry and culture. This book fuses philosophy and the study of home based on many years of extensive research. Richardson looks at how the notion of home, or perhaps the lack of it, can affect identity and in turn the British housing market. This book argues that the concept of 'home' and physical housing are intrinsically linked and that until government and wider society understand the importance of home in relation to housing, the crisis is only likely to get worse.

This book will be essential reading for postgraduate students whose interest is in housing and social policy, as well as appealing to those working in the areas of implementing and changing policy within government and professional spaces.

Joanna Richardson is Professor of Housing and Social Research at De Montfort University. She has previously worked as a housing practitioner for a local authority and a housing association as well as the Chartered Institute of Housing.

Routledge Focus on Housing and Philosophy

Routledge Focus offers both established and early-career academics the flexibility to publish cutting-edge commentary on topical issues, policy-focused research, analytical or theoretical innovations, in-depth case studies or short topics for specialised audiences. The format and speed to market are distinctive. Routledge Focus are 20,000 to 50,000 words and will be published as eBooks and in Hardback as print on demand.

This book series seeks to develop the links between housing and philosophy. It seeks proposals from academics and policy makers on any aspect of philosophy and its relation to housing. This might include ethics, political and social philosophy, aesthetics, as well as logic, epistemology and metaphysics. All proposals would be expected to apply philosophical rigour to the exploration of housing phenomena, whether this be the policy making process, design or the manner in which individuals and communities relate to housing. The series seeks an international and comparative focus and is particularly keen to include innovative and distinctly new approaches to the study of housing.

Please contact Peter King (pjking1960@virginmedia.com) with ideas for book proposals or for further details.

Books in the series

Thinking on Housing
Words, Memories, Use
Peter King

Social Justice in Contemporary Housing
Applying Rawls' Difference Principle
Helen Taylor

Place and Identity
The Performance of Home
Joanna Richardson

Place and Identity
The Performance of Home

Joanna Richardson

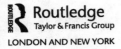

Routledge
Taylor & Francis Group

LONDON AND NEW YORK

First published 2019
by Routledge
2 Park Square, Milton Park, Abingdon, Oxon OX14 4RN

and by Routledge
711 Third Avenue, New York, NY 10017

Routledge is an imprint of the Taylor & Francis Group, an informa business

British Library Cataloguing-in-Publication Data
A catalogue record for this book is available from the British Library

Library of Congress Cataloging-in-Publication Data
A catalog record for this book has been requested

ISBN: 978-0-8153-5204-4 (hbk)
ISBN: 978-1-351-13968-7 (ebk)

Typeset in Times New Roman
by Apex CoVantage, LLC

To my family – for making me feel at home.

Contents

Foreword

Emotion is not a term normally associated with the dry, jargon-infested language of housing and planning policy. This is a book about the emotions and identity that underpin our understanding of home, which is so often obscured by the language of housing units and the minutiae of policy. It is about the emotions – positive and negative – we have towards the places we inhabit and the identity and internal state that is co-created by what Richardson defines as our performance of home. At the same time a duality runs through it. As much as home can be a place of sanctuary, belonging and self-expression, it can also be a place of conflict, violence and, increasingly in the Britain of today, precarity.

The worst housing disaster of modern times, the Grenfell Fire, which killed 72 people and left hundreds homeless, casts a long shadow over the text. In the aftermath of the Fire, the United Nation's Special Rapporteur on the right to adequate housing, Leilani Farha, stated that failing to uphold human rights was, at least in part, the cause of the disaster. She voiced concerns that residents had told her they had been excluded from decisions about housing safety issues before the fire and not been engaged 'in a meaningful way' by the authorities in its aftermath. She was struck by survivors 'feelings of not being heard, of feeling invisible, and not being treated like equal human beings'.

Farha was also concerned that they were stereotyped and discriminated against on the basis that they lived in social housing. Jo Richardson's history of research on the stigmatized experience of home of traveling communities in the UK ensures that there is no better placed observer of today's discriminatory practices, which are now also directed against social housing tenants. Today, these discriminatory practices have entered the mainstream, fueled by the austerity policies disproportionately affecting social housing tenants. The despair and mental health problems that result from frequent evictions are not just the domain of social housing tenants but a large proportion of 'Generation Rent', who pay housing costs well over the 30 per cent of income which is the standard measure across housing studies of 'affordability'.

The housing crisis, symbolized by Grenfell and the discrimination and democratic deficit it brought into stark relief, is the context for any contemporary discussion of housing in the UK. But the multi-disciplinary approach espoused here, drawing on Lefebvre and Doreen Massey's work, also points to new directions which might begin to cast light on a more inclusive approach to housing and the city.

Doreen Massey's concept of 'power geometry', where each individual brings to bear their own set of stories and memories onto each encounter with place creates what Massey describes as 'spatio-temporal events', which co-create place and the city. Lefebvre's work on the production of space and the 'Right to the City' is underpinned by the idea that place is contested and produced by conflicting socio-economic and cultural forces. The impact of the financialization of every aspect of housing and property over the last 30 years has meant that this contestation, which allows multiple voices to be heard, has been superseded by a speculative development industry which is creating mono cultural sterile zones of affluence. At the same time the impact of austerity, combined with the outsourcing and privatization of social housing, is further decimating the housing stock and sending rents in the private sector ever higher.

The consequence is that lower income communities are displaced from their homes to outlying areas where poor conditions proliferate. Ken Loach's film, *I Daniel Blake* portrays the increasingly common experience of families moved to other parts of the country altogether. But what is notable is that while the film was well-received in progressive circles it has not had anything close to the political impact of his seminal 1960s film *Cathy Come Home* which led to national scandal and the formation of the homelessness charity Shelter. Today political discourse is inured to homelessness and eviction and the seeping discrimination against social housing tenants is reflected more accurately in media representations through the proliferation of 'poverty porn' programmes on TV.

Loach's film may have failed to change political discourse but Lefebvre and Massey remain highly influential in academic circles. Doreen Massey was a geographer and Henri Lefebvre a sociologist. As Richardson says, the subject of housing studies is trying to construct an identity for itself but in trying to come to an understanding of home it inevitably draws from a variety of disciplines. These include urban studies, built environment, sociology, geography, cultural studies, architecture, media studies, social psychology, anthropology, criminology and feminist studies, to name but a few and I would suggest this book is essential reading for students in all these areas. There is a lot of rhetoric about the importance of multi-disciplinarity in the Academy at present but in the siloed world of academia it is often difficult to work across disciplines. In this invaluable study Richardson has managed to achieve this and has in the process pointed towards new directions for students, academics and policymakers to build on.

Anna Minton,
London 2018

1 Performing home

An introduction

Home is a cyclical construction of us. We shape home and home shapes us. Home is a feeling, not a structure. We bring home to our house. When we feel 'at home' we can be our true self. But home is not always a fairytale with a fixed happy ending. There are dark corners in our attempt to be 'at home', our house may not protect us – it may indeed feel like a trap.

My aim, in this book, is to build on previous studies of housing and home by opening up a new area for exploration and philosophical reflection – going beyond 'housing as home' and examining instead the intersection of place, identity and performance in our quest for 'home'. The desire for home, the journey to home, the reconstruction of our meaning of home within a space, and our need to locate ourselves – our identity – within the world. These are all aspects of the 'performance' of home. Not limited necessarily to a physical structure, but always linked to a space (geographical or temporal) and a place (physical land or relativity to others). Our home, or our quest for home, is inextricably linked to our identity. The contribution of this book, building on current literature and a range of my own research findings and experiences, is a new frame for thinking about home – adding to the academic debate, offering reflection on political and professional practice for those working in housing and creating a reflective space for all of us currently at, or looking for, home.

Context

Housing – shelter – is one of our basic human needs. Without a place to live, our health and wellbeing is threatened, our sense of connection with community and work is broken. In the longer term, as Maslow (1943) identified, if our basic needs such as shelter are not met, then we cannot go on to fulfil our aspirations and goals and become the best selves we can be. The focus for governments of any political persuasion has been to talk of numbers of housing units that are built, or not. The provision of roofs over heads though is not a satisfactory end point; there is a need to understand further how houses (or other forms of accommodation) become 'home' and to explore the ways in which we view ourselves in connection with home. We must ask what impact home (or the lack thereof) has on our own perceived identity and undertake a more philosophical consideration of what home means. To ensure sufficient provision and management of homes and communities, we need to go beyond bricks and mortar, to examine identity and meaning.

The problem we face is not only an evidenced need for more houses to be built in the right places and at the right price, but a growing number of people who have a roof over their head but who do not have a home, a place within which and from which they can accomplish their goals. Many in Generation Rent are living in high-cost, shared accommodation in the private sector. Some report shoddy landlord practice, revenge evictions, damp, dangerous repairs and pest infestations. Whilst clearly, there are many landlords who do let responsibly, this increasing number of reports from young people show, at the least, a dissatisfaction with the places they currently reside – they are a long way from 'home'.

Exploring and understanding 'home' should not be seen as a philosophical luxury. Of course, without the building of houses, sites, roads, schools and hospitals, then 'home' is not possible. But the built unit is not the end point of home. Some may argue that 'an English man's home is his castle' and that intervention by governments and corporations should stop at the front door. However, as shown by the increasing numbers of reports of poor letting and management practice in a growing private rented sector, there is a need to open the door and offer protection and help where it is needed. We must help people access housing, but then also provide support to create that space or move to another space that can be considered as 'home'. In attempting to understand 'home', we can highlight ways in which government policy, local authority and housing association practice can help support people to accomplish their goals. Debating this is not just a theoretical argument – it can lead to better everyday practice.

The fire at Grenfell Tower, London, in 2017, brought issues of safety, security, housing and home into tragically sharp focus. Over seventy people were eventually named as having been killed by the fire – young, old, men and women from all over the world who had made London their home. Housing policy and debates then must concern themselves with physical structures (and their safety and security) as well as less tangible social and support networks which help to maintain 'home'. Whilst this book argues that 'home' is not only about bricks and mortar, the physical structure of housing is though, vitally important to creating and maintaining home. The personal testimonies of those who lived and lost loved ones in the Grenfell Tower are compelling. The flats – the homes – within the tower, turned from spaces with presumed physical safety and integrity of structure to a death-trap.

Well-maintained houses can be a place of security, but we know the space surrounding house and home can also be one of conflict. This can happen within a space – for example, through domestic violence or other abuse. But it also occurs in the discourse – the debates about housing and home. It can be seen in arguments and objections to new housing development being built which embody the cognitive dissonance around importance of home. It is possible for someone to be heard worrying about the lack of affordable houses in their area for grown-up children starting their own family to be able to rent or buy, but in the following breath object to plans for new development at the bottom of their garden because of the concern on overuse of local doctors, roads and indeed potential negative impact on house prices because of spoilt views. To hold these two thoughts in one head – to understand the importance of home even for our own family and yet to object to new places being built because of the impact on one's own individual dwelling – is challenging but not at all uncommon.

Home can also be inextricably linked with 'ownership' in the political discourse. Getting on the housing ladder invariably means on the ownership ladder. But what does ownership mean in relation to home? It links in many debates to security and to quality, and it also links to wealth – to have an asset base to leverage for the future of yourself and family. However do these characteristics of home have to be in the form of ownership? It is possible to provide security and quality through different rental tenure agreements in the private sector, as found in continental Europe, as well as better regulation of landlords to ensure properties are well maintained – safe and sound. In terms of investing in an asset to leverage, say, social care in old age, there could be better development of alternative financial products that would keep investment as 'safe as houses'. Home shouldn't have to be owned to feel secure, high quality – there need to be alternative ways too for potential future return on investment and savings for individuals and families across generations.

Examining objections to new building can show the appreciation for the need for homes in general, but also the worry about the impact on 'my' home. Such conflict, over use of space and right to 'home', can be extremely problematic for planners and developers – and ultimately for those living in unsatisfactory accommodation who are looking for 'home'. Where such fissures in understanding of home can be explored, there may be more open spaces for negotiation in planning for communities to overcome challenges and conflict.

There is a need for a philosophical debate on housing and home to help contrast with, and provide a challenge to, the overuse of the word 'home' by government, agencies and builders who previously used words like 'units' to describe their constructions. As this book will argue, home is more than bricks and mortar: it is a feeling internalised, represented through emotions, memories, freedom to be our authentic selves, even small objects carried with us to help us carry 'home' in our heart.

This chapter will now go on to introduce, briefly, two key concepts returned to throughout the book – 'home' and 'performing'. Discussed within these two concepts is the notion of 'identity' and the complexity and intersectionality of identities. All of these terms are open to interpretation and personal translation. Whilst this work attempts to discuss meanings and complexity in relation to each and then in relation to our own 'identity' at different points in the book; it is appropriate to note the near impossibility of fixing meaning at one specific point that could be meaningful for all (Laclau and Mouffe, 2001).

Home, identity and performance will all then stretch, change and reset in meaning over time and space and according to individual readers. The challenge is in recognising this, but not shying from the importance of the attempt to understand and recognise such vital concepts as 'home'. This indeed is the key point in this book: if we don't engage with the conflicts inherent in the meaning of 'home', because it is too difficult, this could manifest in the continuing denial of home to many people. If, however, we grapple with 'home' – the ideal outcome would be more sensitive legislation, policy and practice to deliver home.

Home

The book explores different ways that home has meaning. This goes beyond house as home, and includes nuanced intersections of identity and place. Taking the time to investigate the meanings of home is important, because it is such a vital fundamental part of our wellbeing – to feel 'at home'.

In contributing to a framework going beyond 'house as home', definitions are going to be important. This whole book is a discussion on the definition of 'home' as part of the definition of 'us' as performers of our own identities. Home has been the subject of a large variety of texts, for example Despres (1991), Somerville (1997), Chapman and Hockey (1999), Moore (2000), King (2004), Mallett (2004) and Blunt and Dowling (2006) all review and develop this work. This chapter will not undertake a forensic literature review of all the studies and the critiques on home, but it will draw from, and think about some of the key ideas which have emerged.

Despres (1991) undertook a review of the literature on home and outlined categories of meanings of home identified across the studies in the review. They included:

- Home as security and control
- Home as a reflection of one's ideas and values

- Home as acting upon and modifying one's dwelling (achievement and control)
- Home as permanence and continuity
- Home as relationships with family and friends
- Home as centre of activities
- Home as a refuge from the outside world
- Home as indicator of personal status
- Home as material structure (perhaps meaning here as a machine for living)
- Home as a place to own

(Adapted from Despres, 1991, pgs 97–99)

There have been subsequent review articles considering the range of meanings and categories of home. This book takes the argument one step further on thinking about the performance of home. This goes beyond home as a reflection of our identity; but rather on the performance of home we undertake to create and recreate our own identity and place in the world. The complexity and messiness of the meaning of home will be a thread throughout the book. Home is not a singular entity; it is not even bound necessarily within a structure – but can be within us, wherever we are. A secure structure, or place to return to, can help provide the security for home, but it can also entrap us. Home is also in multiple locales, situations, times and scenarios (Massey, 1994). Understanding home is a challenge exactly because it is within us – feelings about home are internalised and therefore difficult to measure and analyse (Ravetz and Turkington, 2011).

This book will weave the many functions of, and dreams for, home – many of these have been touched upon in a body of literature spanning types and categories of home meaning, as drawn together by Despres (1991). Home cannot be seen in isolation from other contexts and locales; indeed Blunt and Dowling (2006) remind us that the meaning of home is constructed within a wider framework of power dynamics.

> *Home as a place and as a spatial imaginary helps to constitute identity whereby people's senses of themselves are related to and produced through lived and metaphorical experiences of home. These identities and homes are, in turn, produced and articulated through relations of power.*

(Blunt and Dowling, 2006, pg 256)

Home is not a vacuum, the inconsistencies, hegemonic patriarchy, inequalities are all brought into home. In exploring the darker side of home, the inconsistency of home, the duty as well as love, the violence as well as the security, then we can learn much more than just looking at idealised norms of what home 'should be'. Chapman (1999) says: '*When we dare to enter the House of Doom we learn much about the ideal home*' (pg 147).

Mallett (2004) highlights the complexities within the built home, the space of home – the interconnections of people within a place. These complexities exist within families, between generations, expectations, identities. A further layer of complexity of relationships can clearly occur in 'home' where there is necessitated sharing with strangers, either because of affordability issues, or characteristics of a housing scheme. Connections between place and people who choose to dwell together and also between people who are strangers and place are complex, but they help us to test the meaning of 'home'.

So, 'home' is complex and difficult to define. We can define 'house' relatively simply though; indeed, Atkinson and Jacobs (2016) say: "*A house is a domestic dwelling, a structure in which people live*" (pg 9). For shorthand a 'house', in this scenario as dwelling, could equally be a bungalow, flat or other bricks and mortar structure in which a household lives. There are many dwelling constructions which are not 'house', but are still constructions, perhaps of home, in different parts of the world – meeting different cultural norms and practices. These will be explored in more detail in an examination of nomadism and home later in the book.

A house, for modern architects like Le Corbusier, was a 'machine for living'. He advocated 'mass building' so that people were able to have these machines to help them live. He makes clear, the importance of the house, and of architecture to deliver machines that support 'living':

> The problem of the house is a problem of the epoch. The equilibrium of society today depends upon it. Architecture has for its first duty, in this period of renewal, that of bringing about a revision of values, a revision of the constituent elements of the house.
>
> (Le Corbusier, 1985 (1927), pg 225)

Looking beyond the house as functional support for living, Bachelard (2014) sees the poetry and the beauty in our dwellings – not solely on a physical aesthetic, but on what they allow us to be:

> if I were asked to name the chief benefit of the house, I should say: the house shelters daydreaming, the house protects the dreamer, the house allows one to dream in peace.
>
> (pg 28)

Gilman (1903) eloquently articulated the complexities of home at the turn of the last century – the duality of love and duty in home and the unvalued work of women in the home. Nevertheless, within that messiness of feeling about home, the security and protection is not lost in that:

> *The time when all men were enemies, when out-of-doors was one promiscuous battlefield, when home, well fortified was the only place on earth where a man could rest in peace, is past, long past. But the **feeling** that home is more secure and protective than anywhere else is not outgrown.*
>
> (Gilman, 1903, pg 27) [original emphasis]

Whilst modernity might have mitigated the need for a fortified home – for the machine we live in – to physically protect us the way we once needed, we can see that the ideas of Bachelard and of Gilman still hold true – there is an emotional and sentimental home, often connected with a physical space or dwelling, but not always necessarily so.

A home goes beyond 'house'. Sometimes, home goes beyond physical construction of any kind – a sound, smell or an image in memory can be 'home' when we need it to be. Close our eyes in an anonymous space – for a moment on a train perhaps – and a piece of music can bring home to mind, a day dream, a photo on our increasingly smart phones. We can look forward to being at home, and for a moment feel at home, even when we're not there – yet. Home is about us, the connections between people and their space:

> *The home, in other words, is a socio-spatial system. It is not reducible either to the social unit of the household, or to the physical unit of the house, for it is the active and reproduced fusion of the two.*
>
> (Saunders and Williams, 1988, pg 83)

We construct home through knowing, experiencing and living. We know the physicality of the space and it becomes part of us the longer we are there (inherently knowing where the stairs begin and end in the dark, how many paces it takes to run to a crying child's bedroom). The longer we are there, the more at home we can feel (Gurney, 1990). We socially and physically construct 'home' (Somerville, 1997), but it also makes and shapes us through our physical experience of living our everyday lives within its boundaries (Dowling and Power, 2012).

Home can be constructed through housing (amongst other things) – but it is a process as well as an entity – reconstructed to reflect changes in our world, identity and context. In talking about the domestic sphere, Blunt (2005) refers to the '*complex entanglements of nature and culture, and of human and nonhuman agency, in shaping the domestic sphere*' (pg 512). Lawson (2006) recognises this complexity in her comparison of home-ownership and housing provision in Australia and the Netherlands – the variety of aspects involved, the different and embedded sets of social relations governing the interaction of people, each with their own view of the world. The social, emotional and physical construction of home is messy and complex, which is why responding to it through policy and legislation is challenging, but also why such a difficult issue should not be left solely to the market.

Home might also be constructed through locales, other than 'our house'. Somerville (1989) critiques the view of Saunders and Williams (1988) that home is the 'crucial medium' for structuring and organising society. He argues that there are other situations for this, such as school and work. I would argue further that when our house, our physical machine for living, works against us, either because of violence from a family member, or because the physicality of the structure doesn't allow us to do the things we want – if it isn't adapted to a disability say – then 'home' may well be school, or the office: a physical space that does allow someone to 'be'. Imagine 'home' for a neglected and hungry child where school offers a breakfast club and the chatter of friends – the feeling of home, for them, is more likely to be situated in the school locale than in the family house. So, there are ways that teachers and employers can also be part of a network of governance and practical help, to support people to feel 'at home', wherever they need that to be.

Woman and home

The glossy magazine *Woman and Home* is read still today, whilst it has modernised to a degree, the very title is reminiscent of a time when 'a woman's place' was in the home. There isn't (unsurprisingly) a title of 'Man and Home' on the magazine racks. Home today is still a heavily gendered space – women are responsible, more than men still, for the work undertaken to make and maintain home – the caring, the tidying and the cooking. Women are still abused, more than men, and by men they know, in the home. Home may still be more heavily a woman's domain, but it is not necessarily always a safe space for women to be.

Gilman (1903) talks of love and duty in the home, it is not only a positive and nurturing space – it can be exhausting and depleting too. Her intention, in writing the work, was to get women outside of the home – to be seen not only through undervalued domestic work, but in society and economy – not trapped only at home.

Whilst my book does not set out as a feminist work on the meaning of home, I do apply a feminist lens, in the literature I've reviewed, in the examples I cite, in the research methods and approaches I've taken during my career, in my understanding – as a woman – of my home.

Complicated and complex home

Home is a precarious and precious thing. Home might also, though, be considered a trap – a place where conflict or abuse might occur and remains hidden. Even where home is relatively safe, it can still feel like a place of work. Our current house may not be 'home' for a variety of reasons – there may be insecurity of tenure which stops residents feeling settled 'at home'. In some circumstances home can be a trap either a place of depletion, violence or isolation. Home may be a safe space from where we can project our authentic self and amplify our life aspirations, but for those without a home, or who are in a site of depletion or isolation, how can one 'perform' the true self within and from the place we currently reside?

For those who do not have a place to give them shelter, people who are roofless, sofa-surfing or sharing a space when they don't want to, then feeling 'at home' can be a distant dream. Alternatively, home may be a place that is 'away' it may be land not shelter – this is certainly a lesson learnt in research with Indigenous groups who are prone to a more nomadic existence and culture. Conversely, for these groups, home may be a historical link with the land and the freedom to travel away and stop in a number of places – it is not a fixed space but a link with land, ancestry and culture.

It has been argued (King, 2017) that home is almost defined by our complacency to it. If we know it is there and take it for granted, then perhaps it truly is home. It is a place from which we can be, not something we manifestly have to think about on a daily basis – until something goes wrong and the thing we take for granted may not be there, or may not work in the way we have come to expect. One can see this very clearly for those who do not have sustainable or secure places to be – they do not have home. This can be on a range from dissatisfaction with neighbours, living in a noisy street, being too far away from family and friends, not enjoying the local school, through to starker consequences of feeling threatened by someone in a house-share, suffering violence or abuse from a family member within the four walls, physically being on the street without shelter or having your mobile accommodation moved on endlessly. Homelessness can be a physical and dangerous reality or a sense of dissatisfaction and a feeling one is unable to be authentic to longer-term ambitions.

If home is a feeling – of security and safety, a place from which to launch into the world every day and fulfil potential – then it is possible to have a house but not a home; indeed it is possible to feel 'at home' outside of bricks and mortar. This does not just refer to those that live in different types of accommodation, but it also brings in those who feel at 'home' with people and outdoor spaces and not with dwelling places. People who have lived on the streets for a long time can feel isolated and not 'at home' when first moved into a shelter because the support that might have been present amongst fellows in the same position is cut off in the new property. In research with Gypsies and Travellers, numerous respondents state feelings of isolation and not being at home when they move into bricks and mortar accommodation – some moving back onto the road – roofless in the sense of being continuously evicted, but perhaps not 'homeless' in the emotional sense, if they are with family again, albeit moved on together along the road.

For those who want to create 'home' – whether that is a fixed dwelling in a place, or the freedom to live according to cultural norms – there are issues that government policy needs to consider about (1) accessing and (2) sustaining home. With homelessness on the rise and the shortage of accommodation, particularly genuinely affordable and secure accommodation, then it is important to explore why 'home' is such a vital space from which to perform our lives. The answer then to 'homelessness' (as opposed to rooflessness) is not solely the building of houses – units. We may need to develop more flexible and adaptive policies and processes to supporting the provision and maintenance of 'home'. This is where conflict can and does arise, when one person's home and sense of place impinges on another – it can be this which causes tensions in planning processes; particularly where home looks markedly different and where assumptions about the qualities of the people who prefer alternative types of 'home' are assumed to be detrimental. In these spaces of conflict, it is so important to define positions and interests carefully and to mediate different and equally valid opinions of what home is, where it should be and what it should look like. Strategic planning for communities of homes is vital to protect different interests, to prevent ad hoc and inappropriate responses to housing need and to ensure appropriate infrastructure and services are in place to help make sure houses can be translated into homes, spaces where we can perform the rest of our lives.

Performing home is a personal process, but that does not mean the policies to provide and manage homes should be done on a presumption of the individualisation of home-making. If it takes a community to raise a child, as the adage goes, then it takes society to help make and support homes. One of the benefits of 'home' is that it is a place to be our authentic selves and to do that it may be necessary to shut out others to create a space for self. But this does not negate the responsibility of society, government, housing providers from the act of supporting home-making and sustaining – for protecting people from harm or depletion within those walls, and for enabling communities to create permeable walls of home, to allow for social human connection.

Performing/performance

There are multiple interpretations of the meaning of performing/ performance. The book interacts with 'performance' in three main ways: (1) performance as doing – a technical undertaking – a task, say, of constructing a home and identity, (2) performance as power – discourse and control as performance of power; and (3) performance as an art form – an act.

Performance as doing

In examining 'home' as a performative space, both within and from the space we call home, it is important to understand what 'home' means, how it links with one's own identity and the ability, power, freedom to act as our authentic selves. If we feel 'at home', we have a stage from which we are enabled to perform the rest of our lives – that is, we feel empowered to be ourselves within home, but also as a place from which to 'launch' into our daily lives: work, school, social interactions with others. That 'stage' – home – from which we can perform, is potentially constructed and reconstructed many times during our lives, and not necessarily because we move physical space. The same building might be constructed as 'home' in different ways depending on a number of external contexts and internal processes. King (2005) talks about housing as a process (a verb) rather than how we might discuss housing in the trade press (a noun) a physical structure of bricks and mortar. Similarly, Jaspal and Breakwell (2014) talk about a process of constructing our own identity – shaped and reshaped by our experiences and our relationships with others. I argue that 'home' is part of our identity – sometimes supporting our authentic performance of self, sometimes a source of conflict and tension distracting us from who we want to be. In examining the meaning of home, it is important to consider the (re)construction and performance of our own identities.

When first discussing 'performance' years ago in the delivery of a conference paper on planning conflict over Gypsy and Traveller sites, I managed to cause some offence to participants in the workshop who thought the 'performance' argument suggested a form of acting or 'fakery'. Indeed the paper did make reference to Silverman's (1982) discussion of 'passing' which broadly explains the necessity for Travellers to 'pass' identity by concealing or denying their heritage, often in a scenario of employment, or to be able to access a particular service where they fear that disclosing their heritage could lead to discrimination. In the case of some planning decisions, I had argued that 'passing' was sometimes the opposite. The requirement to perform one's authentic identity, through the amplification of certain signifying characteristics or behaviours, perceived by society and state (the audience) as 'authentic', is driven by the need and desire to secure appropriate accommodation to call one's home: the need for a particular type of home – a site. Because the planning legislation, for Traveller sites, requires proof of a sufficient amount of travelling for a specific purpose (economic), this is increasingly resulting in the performance (obvious and amplified – performing as theatre) of identity according to perception, as outlined in legislation.

In the above conference paper and the discussion immediately afterwards, I made clear that 'performance' should not necessarily be seen as acting or fakery. Performance (as doing) was a feeling of empowerment (or in adverse circumstances such as in defending a planning application – imperative) to display one's own authentic identity and the links with current or hoped-for 'home'. Increasingly, though, in planning cases for sites – performance has to 'show' – it goes beyond everyday 'doing'. We can perform in the quest to get to home, and then we may perform differently within and from the place we consider to be home. Performance in this sense of 'being oneself' either within or from the home is not acting. It is the opposite of acting, but instead enjoying the space and support to follow authentic aims and goals to fulfil ambitions.

bell hooks (1987) in *Ain't I a Woman?* reminds of the problems inherent in categorising identity on one characteristic, be it race, age, gender – or a perceived role within the home – cook, gardener, mother. Our identities, our authentic selves, are not monochrome and easily definable; they are at an intersection at various points and in different contexts. We will perform our identities in different ways in different spaces, or indeed in the same space. Home is an interesting intersection of our identity where we may amplify or dampen different parts of self at different moments and over time and in diverse spaces within the home.

Performance as power

McKenzie (2001) argues that there is a performance stratum that emerges from power and knowledge (and so takes us on from Foucauldian 'discipline'). His work focuses on three main performances – the efficacy of cultural performance, the efficiency of organisational performance and the challenge of technological performance. He asks us to be critical of performance as power itself:

> who – or what – decides what performance is and who – or what –
> performs that which is decided?

(McKenzie, 2001, pg 16)

So, if we consider that performance builds on 'discipline' as a twenty-first century understanding of power in society, it is important to examine what we mean by power and discursive control. Those who hold that society is essentially co-operative (infinite, variable) maintain that the exercise of power is confined to decision-making alone. Lukes (1974) explains, power is also exercised by control of the political agenda – as much through keeping issues away from decision-making, as through dominating the decision-making process.

Home-making, building and sustaining 'home', is kept out of the neo-liberal political arena. Power can be exercised to exclude issues from the agenda, and in housing policy, the threshold of the home is the frontier which is seldom crossed. The way that government 'performs' in this arena is to use 'home' as an empty signifier (Laclau and Mouffe, 2001) in housing discourse to make it appear that there is sufficient support through policy. However, what is actually delivered (or not) is a set number of houses (or 'units') oftentimes with a dearth of supporting infrastructure or services as a result of poorly set or implemented planning gain agreements with developers.

If we see performance as power – power to build houses or to exclude home-making from politics, power to deny home to others for fear of the impact on 'my' home, and power to be one's authentic self within and from 'home' – then performance can be a useful construct for further examination of what home means to me, you, all of us. It can help untangle and re-tangle meanings and constructions of meaning, in a way that takes us beyond bricks and mortar and looks at housing, as home, in the round of what it allows us to do and achieve in our lives.

Performance as art

The domestic space is a rich seam to mine for artistic expression, a huge amount of novels, plays, television and radio dramas are based on the domestic space. From Emin's (1998) *My Bed*, through many light-hearted 'Aga sagas' or grittier 'Kitchen Sink dramas', to the more troubling reflection on the performance of making of home even in the most awful circumstances of kidnap and control, such as we find in the book *Room* by Donahue (2010) – 'home' and the creation and maintenance of home (and identity), is the site of many artistic performances, literary and art works.

However, the very act of living, of making home, is also performed. So not the representation of domestic life and the creation of 'home' on the page or canvas; but creation of home as performance – sometimes as an artistic piece, sometimes also as activist protest, sometimes both. Orlek (2017) debates performance as 'stealth architecture' and examines two residential performances. The first of these is 'Ikea Disobedients' where everyday activities were performed amongst improperly assembled furniture – the audience were invited to participate in these interactions. The second was 'EXYT', which was a 'temporary architecture project' with people living and sleeping in unusual spaces, such as a swimming pool (Orlek, 2017, pgs 184–185).

There are also examples of an overlap between life as art and art as life. Performances based on the domestic (re)creation of home can be difficult to distinguish from the artistic interpretation of performance as power – or protest through occupation; or indeed art as meanwhile use of vacant residential space. In the Dale Farm protest, there was significant interpretation of the motives of protestors and in one iconic photograph from the site, was of a Traveller in front of a fire, holding a cross aloft – she was not a resident, but a protestor occupying the site to prevent eviction; this was performance as power, reinterpreted through photographs in the media as an artistic performance (see further Richardson, 2016, pg 187).

The use of performance art as meanwhile use of domestic space can be seen in the highly successful *Shuffle* festival. I was undertaking a piece of research looking at community land trusts in 2013/14 and was fortunate to meet and talk with members of the East London Community Land Trust who were working with the Mayor and other key housing and local authority partners to develop St Clements Hospital for housing for the community. During the development of the site, and to make best meanwhile use of space and involve the local community in the performance of the space during planning and development, the *Shuffle* festival was created. The film-maker Danny Boyle curated the festival, which included a play by local school students, art installations, dances and film showings. The festival itself has been repeated, but it was in the process and planning of the performances, and the preparation of what was effectively a development site, in order to welcome the community – that was part of the 'performance' of creating 'home' for the East London residents.

'Fake news' as Donald Trump would have it, has been reported in a number of documentaries focusing on habitat and home in recent years – from sequence editing to outright creative scene-building in anthropological and nature programmes. We saw this when Millard's (2018) documentary exposed the fact that tribal tree-houses had been built at the behest of previous documentary teams, to fill in the spaces of the imaginary perceptions the viewers might have of forest tribes. Homes were literally created for the TV, to physically try and demonstrate the residents as more magical and mysterious, more 'authentic' than their real housing and modern ways would show. Higson (1984) discusses the flipside of the phenomenon – housing creating people, as an issue in non-documentary TV. The kitchen sink dramas, such as Coronation Street and others – whilst fictitious, attempted to portray 'real life', but with the place imbuing the characters with a perceived identity – Northern 'grit'. In the construction of identity through place, as an aspect of TV dramas, Higson (1984) noted that '*place becomes a signifier of character, a metaphor for the state of mind of the protagonists*' (pg 3).

Expectations are put upon residents in certain places to 'act' in a certain way – perhaps to be 'traditional' (old-fashioned) in a positive and rose-tinted view of the world. Legislation and policy literally require some groups to act-perform in a way to meet imagined expectations – Travellers must travel to be 'real'. As well as us defining home – home defines us. This can have an adverse impact when home (as shown in artistic performance) imbues the human residents with negative perceived characteristics, which are then met with hostility or indifference by an audience that thinks this characterisation is authentic and real in everyday life.

In considering home as performance in the artistic sense, we can see home sometimes as a protagonist – a sinister character (a trap), or a saviour (forever happy). Sometimes, it is the background narrator – explaining, but at the same time defining and redefining human characters. Home changes in meaning, in performance as a protagonist, narrator, shaper or prisoner, in context and time; it can, if it is a complacent but complicated thing, be neither trap nor saviour – it can be us, as we are, now in this moment.

What next?

In attempting to understand 'home', this book will include exploration of different types of home – not just bricks and mortar. It will examine home as a potential site of conflict and depletion and point to the need for policy to help negotiate isolation and marginalisation. The book also attempts to analyse how we sometimes see our own home as precious and vital to our own well-being whilst at the same time objecting and preventing others from accessing their own home. Whilst the book is intended as a 'think piece' its aim is not only to reflect, but also to project potential pathways to improved policy and practice as a result of understanding home better.

This book is philosophical in nature, but it will draw from experience and research in practice to exemplify key points. This is a personal topic with different meanings, as discussed earlier. My interest in working in and writing about housing comes from a variety of experiences. My understanding of the importance of 'home' was brought into stark view many years ago (1991) during a school project for a month in New York volunteering to help homeless people – the impression that was imprinted during that time underpinned a deep sense of the importance of housing and home. What followed was a career in housing practice and policy before falling into academia. Throughout the decades that followed, the meaning of 'home' and the vital need for adequate, secure and sustainable housing as the first step to home-making has remained a central tenet of my work.

In this piece, there will be a range of research projects which will be drawn from to illustrate key points. These include small evaluative con-sultancy research assignments on various schemes, accommodation assess-ments and projects – some previously completed and some ongoing. Also included, are lessons learnt in other research, funded variously by AHRC, ESRC and JRF. In other words, this philosophical book is underpinned by lessons learnt from years of practice and research and it aims to draw from those experiences to attempt to understand the meaning of 'home' and how that understanding can help us – academics, policy makers and practitioners to support people to feel 'at home'.

The book is also inter-disciplinary – housing studies has been in the pro-cess of trying to construct its own identity and platform – to be of itself a discipline. Housing studies though offers a space for a variety of ideas to intersect, just as home offers an intersection for a range of performances. I will, therefore, draw from a variety of disciplines including built environ-ment, urban studies, geography, cultural studies, architecture, media studies, anthropology, social psychology and feminist studies, for example, which have made contributions to our understanding of home.

Looking ahead to the chapters that follow, there is a breadth of concepts and ideas on place, space, identity and negotiation of conflict, but which wrap around the central themes of 'performing home'.

In the next chapter (2), *'Feeling at home'*, the emotionomics of home will be examined by looking at the intersection of place and identity. Lefeb-vre's (1991) approach to perceptions of space and place is instructive at this point. Place (and home) looks different through varying sets of eyes, and as Massey (2005) shows is inextricably bound up in identity. Planners and citizens will see space differently and so the end use of a place will change from concept on paper, to reality, and over time. There is of course a need for home to physically support us. Part of the complacency of home is not having to count the number of stairs or feel around for a light switch – if it is home, then we know. Where home can become a physical trap is when needs change with age, disability or the addition of new members of the family in a space that is too small for everyone's needs. As noted by the chapter title, feeling 'at home' is inherently emotional. Our identity(ies) are at an intersection at home as much as they are beyond the threshold. Some of that is related to what goes on within – the people we share our home, and our neighbouring spaces, with; but some is from outside – insecurity of the space itself.

Chapter 3, *'Protecting home'* looks further at the emotional attachment to home and the space around it. The question will be asked: is home a site of restoration or depletion? As suggested earlier, the space one currently lives in might not always be a place to 'recharge the batteries' – it could feel like a trap – a place of conflict possibly as a result of neighbour nuisance, domestic violence or abuse. The darker side of home can be a site of depletion through duties of social reproduction (Gilman, 1903; Rai et al., 2013). For women particularly, but not exclusively, home can be another job 'to do' on return from the office, it is less a place of rest and recuperation and perhaps more one of domestic work and child care. This chapter will also look at conflict and negotiation in perceiving, living-in and protecting 'home'. The need to protect home and the family within is a strong urge, which can manifest in planned spaces to amplify security and protection – such as gated communities. In some ways, there is an urge to protect the value of home. If, for example, a new proposed development is feared to impact on house prices, or spoil the view, or decrease easy access to existing services then existing residents in an area may object to plans. A knee-jerk response is to label objectors as NIMBY, but this further embeds positions, rather than seeking to understand interests; and it does not help negotiate out of conflict. It is only in understanding 'interests', which can stem from the meaning of home, that arguments can start to be understood and resolved.

Following on from the debate on conflict over, and protection of, 'home', chapter 4 *'Home screen'* will tease out ideas over the supposed privacy of home that is so hard-fought. Does the threshold of the doorway denote the line between public and private? Since the evolution of information and communication technology, and the development of social media platforms along with better online connectivity in many areas, there has been a blurring of public and private that does not stop at the door. Increasingly, we are seeing the performance of home online with Facebook – representations of a happy home and highly functioning family for thousands to see. In this virtual world, filters are applied to make visual representations of one's home and oneself look more appealing, in this sense – less of a performance and more of an act; but in so doing perhaps making our identity less authentic and our house less of our home. Does the world online mean that our homes are screens that project or protect us?

'Precarious Home' – chapter 5 – examines notions around the precarity of home. With increasing numbers of people who are homeless and living on the street, and more still – many from Generation Rent – living in unsatisfactory, often shared, sometimes dangerous dwellings, the precariousness of home is never more evident. Additionally, 'home' is often discussed in the same breath as 'ownership' – one is seen to truly, finally, have a home when it is owned rather than rented. With the proportional decline in owner occupation and the increase in the private rented sector, the younger generation are even further from 'home' – trapped, for some, in an unwanted

extended childhood back living with parents, feeling unable to move on and create their own families – constrained by lower wages and higher house and living prices. The unaffordability of a secure and decent home is seen most starkly in the mountain (rather than ladder) to climb for the home-ownership goal, but it is also evident in the rented sector with many properties out of reach. Home is not just an individual product, where good governance stops at the front door. There is a need for government and societal mediation of the performance of home to (a) support people to access it in the first place and (b) to mediate conflict of home within four walls, between people and places.

In Chapter 6, '*Home and away*', it is argued again that home is more than the bricks and mortar of a house – it holds different meanings. For some, home is a base from which to travel from. Some of the arguments around provision of Gypsy-Traveller sites and the misrepresentation of that culture relate to different imaginings of 'home'. One sometimes hears the refrain – 'if they're Travellers why don't they travel?' in planning objection arguments. Nomadism is a part of cultural heritage rather than necessarily everyday practice and often, given the chance of a permanent base from which they can travel – Gypsy-Travellers would like to do just that. When 'home' as a base has to be fought over though, the freedom to travel from and back to 'home' can seem like a distant dream. Conversely, 'home' to Gypsy-Travellers may be a series of traditional spaces on a centuries-old route used by generations. There may be favourite places based on memories, or on current welcome, but 'home' is the journey and the family, and not necessarily just the place. Again, and increasingly with public space protection orders, urban and rural spaces are securitised, common land is fenced, deep verges are bunded-off. This is not just an issue for Gypsies and Travellers in England – it is evident for Indigenous communities across the globe (and indeed as a result of urban securitisation resulting in 'homeless spikes' it can have a far-reaching effect on a large number of people). 'Home' may be linked to a piece of land, or a constellation in the sky, to the feeling of custodianship and nature – it is not easily defined or planned for, does not sit within planning boundaries or political jurisdictions, and does not necessarily make sense to people who live in houses.

'*Home is in the heart*' questions how home might be in us, rather than us in home. Our identity and authentic self are wrapped up in home – either our current dwelling if that 'feels like home' or some other place or time. It was suggested earlier, that home isn't always in our house. For various reasons 'home' may be more authentically performed in alternative locales – like school or work. If work is home – the impact, when there are changes in workplace values and visions, are significant on our sense of self and identity. Chapter 7 reflects on the values of working in the social housing sector – the tussle between head and heart of the sector – and the effect of changing values and practices on those working in the sector. Trinkets relating to 'home' or culture, held with us, can help to remember who we are to reinforce our authentic identity and, where we don't live 'at home' in our current dwelling place, can make life more bearable. Notions of identity, which were introduced in chapters two and three, are examined again in this chapter, to suggest that, in addition to home being an intersection for our identity(ies) it can also be with us, represented by proxy objects and memories that help to keep 'home' alive.

The concluding chapter, '*Going Home*', clarifies the contribution of the book in going beyond 'house as home' and thinking of the 'home in us' – the intersection of place and identity. Home goes beyond bricks and mortar – it is feeling, family, roots, history, culture, stage, screen, shelter, self, freedom and trap. In concluding, this chapter will underline the support that is needed from government and society, the understanding of different concepts and meanings of home that should be reflected on – in order that the ambitions to 'make a home' can be more widely achieved. I suggest a framework of conditions necessary for creating home and for supporting home. I have drawn on experience decades working in and with the social housing sector (in practice, policy and academia) to outline ways in which we can all help – community, government, housing practitioners and local politicians – to contribute and support people in creating and maintaining home – wherever and whenever that might be. I believe that in better understanding 'home' we should be better equipped to reframe housing politics, policy and practice for the future.

2 Feeling at home
Intersections of place and identity

Introduction

Home goes beyond a house; it goes beyond dwelling as a noun and moves to dwelling as a verb – as being. 'Home' is an emotional yet politicised and emptied word in public policy discourse. 'Homes for All' is national government policy, but it doesn't embed in action as a human right – there aren't homes for all resulting from the rhetoric. In this chapter, I try to bring together 'house' and 'home' in a discussion on the intersection of place and identity.

The evidence of a housing shortage is clear (for example: longer waiting lists for social housing, increased levels of homelessness, young adults returning to parental homes, fewer and fewer young people accessing the owner-occupied market and harrowing stories from 'Generation Rent'). The rational response in the face of this, surely, is to build more houses. But it's complicated. There is more at stake in the discourse on development planning, than a purely rational response to market information. There are conflicting views within communities, indeed within families, on the response to planning applications to build more homes. A couple approaching retirement who own their home may, at the same time, be wishing for an increase in the value of their capital asset but yet mourn the lack of affordable housing available locally for their adult children to move into. They fear that a planning application for more houses on the edge of their village will affect the value of their current home, but in the same head space, they understand more affordable local housing may be the solution to their wider family's housing need.

Home is not just another asset. Yes, it may also be a physical construction that has a value ascribed to it by a market shaped by supply and demand. However, our relationship with our home, and indeed with the market, is more complex than it is with other assets we may own. Economics has increasingly engaged with the irrational responses to data that form part of decision-making and understanding of social phenomena (Levitt and

Dubner, 2005) and it is important that the emotional economics of housing and planning are also explored in more depth.

Do we find rest at home, or do we have to work to create it? Do we love or sometimes even hate home? The answer is all of these things – at different times in the day, the week, the year, our lives – home supports or exhausts us in different ways. The experience of home is still gendered, as it was in the time of Gilman's (1903) critique. Exploring notions of self and identity at the intersection of home, it can be seen that home is not always a place to 'recharge the batteries'.

Planning for, and living in, homes, is an emotional process that includes conflict in the same individual's thought processes, let alone within and between communities. Emotions in and about home should be considered, to try to move the debate on from rational market arguments of efficiency, house value, need and demand to more of a 'social home emotionomics' approach. Negotiating the outfall from the emotionomics within the home, but also more widely in the community about 'home', is discussed further in Chapter 3, but touched on here.

Constructing identity

The complexities of identity through a defining set of characteristics perceived by individuals, groups and others is discussed by Bordieu (1998) in his explanation of 'habitus':

> *The habitus is this generative and unifying principle which retranslates the intrinsic and relational characteristics of a position into a unitary lifestyle, that is, a unitary set of choices of persons, goods, practices . . . habitus are differentiated, but they are also differentiating . . . But the essential point is that, when perceived through these social categories of perception, these principles of vision and division, the differences in practices, in the goods possessed, or in the opinions expressed become symbolic differences and constitute a veritable language.*
>
> (Bordieu, 1998, pg 8)

So our habitus is our language of home. It is comprised of ideas, expressions and possessions: reflecting our identity. Our homes are differentiated – different from one another, but also differentiating – defining us and our identities and placing us in relation to one another. We make home and home makes us. And for what purpose? Identities through home intersect in various locale to different ends. There is no singular purpose to home, if we go beyond the housing as home paradigm. Home may reflect identity and individual hopes in a variety of ways – going beyond shelter, beyond capital investment for future return. Our different and unique identities create different senses of home. We are constantly recreating our dwelling:

> *The proper dwelling plight lies in this, that mortals ever search anew*
> *for the essence of dwelling, that they must ever learn to dwell.*
>
> (Heidegger, 1993, pg 363)

This language of identity and difference, uniqueness, requiring particular treatment is problematic when each one of our identities includes a number of constructions of self (both perceived by us, and by 'them') which intersect. Identity politics, particularly as spaces within which power can dominate and marginalise, can be problematic (Crenshaw, 1991; Butler, 1999).

We are more than one identity label. Singular identity, based on gender or race, or religion or age, has served to highlight needs of particular groups within a frame of social equality and justice. But it has also neglected the complexity of identity, the interrelations between us and place, the connections that create home.

Rather than protection from inequality, for women, home can be a mirror held up to society, magnifying the imbalances in this private space behind closed doors. Home is gendered – there is an impact on our authentic identity even when in the 'protection' of home. Lloyd and Johnson (2004) also note the difference between the 'dream' of home and the gendered and class-based contradictory reality:

> *This discourse of the dream home resolved lived contradictions in the*
> *national imaginary, particularly for women, and expressed a new desire*
> *for harmony between women's and men's spheres in the discourse of*
> *family togetherness. This togetherness was important not just in gender*
> *terms, but also in categories of class. The reorganisation of the flows*
> *between previously carefully policed boundaries – between clean and*
> *dirty areas and visible and invisible activities – reverses earlier forms*
> *of domestic organisation identified with the emergence of the middle*
> *class in the early 19th century.*
>
> (Lloyd and Johnson, 2004, pg 262)

Singular constructions of identity, and difference, are problematic in constructing society as home for groups who are seen to be 'other'. This has been something I've noticed in my work over the last two decades in researching the accommodation needs of Gypsies and Travellers. They are constructed, through the lens of 'other' as not fitting in with our societal concepts of home – not belonging.

Visoka (2018) suggests that a fluid approach to identity is helpful, in order to *'capture the performativity and temporality of identities'* (pg 75). Indeed, Jenkins (2008) discusses the orientation of identity within a group, through a reflection of self-reference. There are challenges within, on how groups reflect and project group identity, which then impacts on their own individual identity. Tajfel's (1981) work on social identity, highlights the importance of group identity on self:

> *that part of an individual's self-concept which derives from his knowledge of his membership of a social group (or groups) together with the value and emotional significance attached to that membership.*
>
> (Tajfel, 1981, pg 255)

If group identity is so importantly reflected in our own self-identity, then it can become problematic when we are separated from the wider group. Separation might be on a conceptual level – feeling unable to perform everyday ritual activities which reflect belonging to a group; or it might be on a physical level – separated by being in singular units of accommodation, not in proximity to kith and kin.

I remember being at a seminar, listening to a prominent Gypsy-Traveller woman, telling us about a speech she had given at another conference. "I was telling them' [settled people/ non Gypsy-Travellers]", she said, "about how wonderful it was to live next to your mother, father, sisters, brothers, uncles and aunties, grandparents and cousins – doors open, always there. And I noticed the looks of horror and incomprehension on their faces", she concluded to large laughs from fellow conference goers. In a funny anecdote, the speaker, had highlighted the difference in ideal home for different groups – for herself and other members of Gypsy and Traveller communities, this was characterised as wanting to be in very close proximity to the wider family, with doors wide open. For 'settled' people, the ideal home was characterised, through the incomprehension and the laughs at the conference, as being private, closed doors as refuge, possibly from the wider family as well as 'strangers'.

To show one's identity – either an authentic attempt at being and outwardly presenting oneself, or through an act of 'passing', individually or as part of a social identity in a group – is a performance. Goffman talked about this in his (1959) work on presentation of self:

> *A status, a position, a social place is not a material thing, to be possessed and then displayed; it is a pattern of appropriate conduct, coherent, embellished and well-articulated. Performed with ease or*

clumsiness, awareness or not, guile or good faith, it is none the less something that must be realized.

(Goffman, 1959, pg 81)

Housing as a verb rather than a noun denotes a journey of construction and re-creation. In a similar vein, identity might also be thought of as a journey or a process.

Breakwell (2014) also explicitly talks about a process of identity:

IPT [Identity Process Theory] *argues that the individual engages, consciously or unconsciously in a dynamic process of constructing an identity and that this process is continual. Every new experience is interpreted in relation to the existing identity content and evaluation. Each new experience could potentially call into question the legitimacy of the existing identity structure . . .*

(Breakwell, 2014, pg 118)

We need to consider identity as a process, in relation to social group, context, economy and politics. This process of identity formation and renewal, might be incremental and slight, or in seismic shifts in response to singular events or crises. Home is complex because of the intersections of our own identity as individual and group, and the further intersection of that with our space and place. We need privacy, but connectedness, a space to be alone, but also with others, a place to demonstrate our own unique identity. But we also need a place to construct the shared identity of family within or the shared identity with others, out-with the physical space of house as home.

By bringing cultural constructs to the study of self-concept, this paradigm has made clear that there are multiple self-goals – to be part of and connect with others and to be unique and distinct from others.

(Oyserman, 2004, pg 17)

Aboriginal people and other Indigenous communities can help us see the importance of identity and place so intertwined. The history of Australia has predominantly been presented through the lens of white men; but more recently voices of Aboriginal women have started to disrupt the received wisdom. Having not even been recognised as human inhabitants (the original doctrine of terra nullius) of the land they'd called home for thousands of years, Aboriginal people have withstood physical and cultural destruction, and in the face of adversity, still now, are continuing to tell the story of their history, place and identity and to fight for their rights to the land (Weedon, 2004). This will be explored more later in the

book in Chapter 6 on 'Home and away' – going beyond the physical construct of house to examine nomadism and home. But the understanding
of Aboriginal identity construction with place is an important reflection
at this point.

Understanding 'place'

> To travel between places is to move between collections of trajectories
> and to reinsert yourself in the ones to which you relate. Arrived at work,
> in Milton Keynes, I re-join debates, teams meeting to discuss teaching,
> a whole cartography of correspondence, ongoing conversations, pick up
> where I left off the last time I was 'here'. Back in London at night I
> emerge into the energising bedlam of Euston Station and go through the
> same process again. Another place, another set of stories . . . Places not
> as points or areas on maps, but as integrations of space and time, as
> spatio-temporal events.
>
> (Massey, 2005, pg 131)

We are not only consumers of space, but also creators and re-creators of
'place' as we move through time and physical space, capturing moments,
glimpses of views, imaginings of people and objects. Places are porous
networks of social relations and the 'power geometry' debated by Massey,
emphasised how groups and individuals are differently positioned within
these porous networks. People define themselves in terms of 'place' and
understand their position within this network. Place is both empowerment
and disempowerment, depending on the identity and perceived identity of
the individuals and groups interacting with it.

Lefebvre's (1991) framing of a 'Triad of Space' debates connections,
from the point of view of an individual's perception of the realms of space.
Lefebvre discusses the need for interconnectedness between 'lived, real
and perceived realms'. He makes very clear that this concept should not be
viewed in the abstract, if its importance is to be retained:

> That the lived, conceived and perceived realms should be intercon-
> nected, so that the 'subject', the individual member of a given social
> group may move from one to another without confusion – so much is a
> logical necessity. Whether they constitute a coherent whole is another
> matter. They probably do in favourable circumstances, when a common
> language, a consensus and a code can be established.
>
> (Lefebvre, 1991, pg 40)

Favourable circumstances for interconnectedness between these realms certainly do not exist in the process and debate surrounding planning policy for

non- traditional housing, such as Gypsy and Traveller sites, or for contentious developments of, for example, wind farms or recycling plants. One cannot see evidence of a common language, code or consensus between different groups and individuals living in a particular geographical area and therefore it is unlikely that Lefebvre's conceptual triad can be anything but abstract in the realm of planning policy and decision-making for the use of space in housing provision. Indeed the language surrounding debate on providing non-traditional housing is divided and divisive, as previous research on the use of discourse to control Gypsy and Traveller issues has shown (Richardson, 2006).

Gentrification and place marketing have reduced some spaces, on the surface, to blandness and sameness. Cosslett (2015) suggests gentrified London is 'sterile and dull' as a result of the 'triumph of the hive mind'. Mahdawi (2015) pokes fun at the attempt by business improvement districts and developers to bring in American-style place marketing 'zones' and 'quarters' – *"Let's meet in Midtown!" said no one in London, ever* (Mahdawi, 2015). People and places need to rebel against the hegemony of beige gentrification, in the face of some areas of London being the sole preserve of rich individuals and businesses (Minton, 2017) and with common spaces increasingly out of the reach of city residents (Minton, 2009). Places in cities, and in towns and villages are sites of protest as well as dwelling (Richardson, 2016). Hostile architecture increasingly dictates the use of formerly shared spaces, leaving fewer places for homeless people to sleep, stopping Gypsies from travelling through traditional routes, preventing people from being in a place. Harvey (2013) refers to the right to the city and the need for a revolution and Vasudevan (2017) reminds us of the history of squatting – a performance of protest as well as creation of home.

Spaces and places are contradictory. And we know this must be so from our own interactions as humans constructing and consuming our own home. But also for those working in housing and planning professions, seeing how planned spaces, planned policies and planned management processes change as we live those plans and see them reconstructed to work in newly created and recreated realities. Easthope (2004) underlines the importance of discovering home as an 'important place'. She refers to the significance of interconnectedness in understanding home:

> *understanding homes as particularly significant places means that housing researchers who are concerned with home must look beyond the house in their investigations, since homes (like all places) are nodes in networks of social relations. In order to understand home, we need to understand these networks.*

(Easthope, 2004, pg 136)

The home is a locale of intersecting plans, ideas and power relations. It is particularly important for those working in policy and practice not to take 'home' as a taken for granted physical construction, but instead to keep in mind the intersection of power and emotions at play.

In attempting to define place and space, de Certau (1988) clarifies: "In short, *space is a practiced place*" (pg 117). Place and space cannot be abstract in the sense-making of home, each are made through interaction with people. Tuan (1977) contends that space is more abstract than place, which turns de Certau (1988) on its head. My feeling is that, by inhabiting space and connecting with self, we create place through personal perspective and experience. Place is less abstract than space, as it positions me geographically, temporally, socially with other people and objects.

Land is clearly an important physical contribution to 'place'. So much is obvious, but it is a difficult balance between land and the built environment. The spirit of a place can be amplified through people, chatter, the buzz of traffic, music, food cooking, sirens blaring in a city. Or, mud squelching, bird singing, grass rustling, rain dropping in the countryside. In both, the spirit is felt by those residing or visiting that space, meeting others there (humans or animals), connecting with the land under our feet, remembering generations past – in that place.

in our ever-more internationalised, corporatized, mediated and de-individualised world, the spirit of a place, the sum of the meeting of people and land, remains of vital importance.

(Dee, 2018, pg 12)

The relationship between us and place is a circular, self-defining process. I make sense of my place, and my place redefines me. At home, I feel I can be myself, I can be 'complacent' (King, 2017) about home, because it is mine and it's there; but there are moments, interactions with people or objects, or the view from the window that make me objectively appreciate the place, my home. This is my everyday understanding of Bordieu's (1998) 'habitus' – the link between place and self: home.

The architecture of spaces and places is important in helping us to construct feelings of safety and security. Kemsley and Platt (2012) note how enclosed structures (single rooms, caves, hidey holes) can help '. . . *transform us from anxious victims to secure observers*' (pg 83). Bernheimer (2017) underlines the wellbeing effects of our surroundings in three realms – physical, functional and psychological. This book argues that good housing can provide physical and functional wellbeing, but I argue that for psychological wellbeing, a person needs to feel 'at home'.

Place can be inclusionary or exclusionary on a whim, depending on who is travelling through the place, or residing in a place, what they are doing and how they are being. Massey (2005) discusses immigration and place with a story about an 'immigrant boulder' discovered in Hamburg by engineers working on the bed of the River Elbe. The boulder made the news and was soon used in place marketing advertisements, it was taken to people's hearts in Hamburg. But scientists found the boulder was not a native environmental feature but had been pushed by ice thousands of years ago – it was labelled 'Hamburg's oldest immigrant', which prompted Massey to ask: *"How long do you have to have been here to be local?"* (Massey, 2005, pg 149). In 2018, the scandal of the treatment by the British government of the Windrush migrants from the 1950s to the 1970s came to a head in political and media discourse. People who had come to school here, married, worked, had children and grandchildren, were finding that they didn't have the right 'paperwork' and were receiving disturbing documentation threatening deportation. They would rightly have had a sense of rootedness (Tuan, 1977) in Britain, even a sense of complacency in a country they had come to feel as home; only to have that sense of place, that sense of British identity disrupted, and 'home' threatened, because of 'paperwork'.

Local, and the sense of belonging to a specific part of the world, is an important concept in how we see ourselves, our place – and also how others see us. 'Local' can be seen as parochial, strange, inward-looking (as amusingly portrayed in their television show, by the 'League of Gentlemen' through the fictitious Royston Vasey, – for *local* people). 'Local' can vary in scale – in the Brexit debate, local became national in the discourse of protecting 'our borders'. Local is somewhere though, it is not global – however through online networks the local and the global can come together to be 'glocal'; particularly in protest. Goodhart (2017) sums up the issue of 'local' in a reflection on populist politics and the discourse around the Brexit referendum. He refers to two 'tribes' in Britain – the 'Anywheres' (degree educated and mobile) who in the majority voted to remain, and the 'Somewheres' (working class, particularly in the North) who voted to leave. The Somewheres were local, felt their place under threat – perhaps from immigrants, perhaps from a lack of employment or investment in infrastructure, or an absence of a reflection of who they thought they were – what their place looked like, in the Westminster political and media mirror. Ironically, some of the 'Somewhere' communities and places were exactly the spots where European Union funds had been invested. The less well-off 'Somewhere' communities may be seen as marginal and liminal spaces (Richardson, 2017a; Shields, 1991) in the eyes of government and media.

The perception of those living in 'Somewhere' communities may be different, in view and outlook from a closer perspective, seeing their place as 'home' – connected to their identity with that space. But this binary debate of 'Somewheres' and 'Anywheres' can be divisive and open to caricature – at some point, we feel our identity connect with other people in a place (geographical, temporal) and in that moment (even if it is a distant nostalgic memory) it is home.

Nurturing and supportive home

Homemaking is not a one-way process where people simply appropriate objects, furnishings, colours and textures to achieve feelings of homeyness. Rather it is a multi-directional relation where the materiality of the house also shapes and potentially surprises, disturbs and alters residents' sense of home.

(Dowling and Power, 2012, pg 77)

The stage from which we perform – home – must be adapted to our physical needs. We grow to instinctively know our home, not have to count the stairs, or where the light switch is. For older people or disabled people there is a need for adaptations to allow home to be that stage and not to become a trap. We know that meaning of home becomes stronger, the longer we are there (Gurney, 1990). For older people who have been in their homes for very many years, the emotional knowing of home may not be reflected in the physicality of the house – what was once ten paces across the room, becomes 20 shuffling steps, the windows too far to reach, the sockets too low, the stairs too much. How do we retain 'home' when the house starts to work against us? We create home, and home shapes us – it is necessary in some cases to recreate home so it continues to support rather than hinder our living.

Home can become a trap for a person who has been injured and becomes physically disabled from using their accommodation as a 'machine for living', as they used to. Seeing the transformation that adaptations can bring, for example through having adjustable kitchen counter top heights to ensure a disabled young man can reach for a glass of milk or help his Mum, like he used to, in preparing meals from his wheelchair – it is liberating. At times like this, it is perfectly obvious that a social model of disability (with the onus on wider society) rather than a medical model (with the onus on the physical abilities of the person) is so important in policy and law making, as well as in design and build of our locales – home, school and work. Adapted spaces can nurture and support – they can be, again, the platform or stage from which we can perform our lives.

For older people, who find the house is too big, the garden difficult to maintain, the stairs challenging to climb and the local shops increasingly far away, then sometimes leaving home is the only option to keep someone physically safe. Steward (2000) notes the need for a more sociological perspective of home when considering the needs of disabled people. In their review, Roy et al. (2018) advocated for homes to be adapted where possible, but they recognised there were still steps that could be taken to help recreate home, in the event an older person had to move.

> *emphasizes the importance of adapting dwellings and communities to older adults wishing to stay at home in the residential environment that they know and value. It also pushes us to reconsider how we design alternative housing for frail older adults . . . alternative housing should also integrate meaning-of-home considerations that could help older adults adapt to their new dwelling and rebuild their feeling of being-at-home.*

(Roy et al., 2018, pg 26)

Designing-in 'feeling-at-home' is vital for older people, worried that they may lose that sense of the world and their lives. I remember in the late 1990s, for my job at the Chartered Institute of Housing, visiting a small new housing development built by a specialist registered social landlord for Black and Minority Ethnic Elders. The architects had designed the place so the communal spaces felt like a neighbourhood, with corridors as 'streets', vibrant art work – not a hint of beige. Doors to rooms were like front doors so there could be a feeling of self-contained 'home' for privacy. At the time of my visit, the cooking smells were delicious and flavoursome and some of the residents were involved in the meal preparation. It was one of the most joyous visits to an older persons' housing scheme that I have ever made in my housing practice career. The key seemed to be connection – between the residents themselves, with the professionals supporting them, with the memories evoked by the design of the place and the everyday involvement in meal preparation, sometimes with recipes 'from home'.

Sometimes, connection between people and home needs to look beyond peers and, particularly for older people, design in inter-generational contact. Despres and Lord (2005) advocate the consideration of 'accessory apartments' in older person residences, so that 'inter-generational experiences' can occur (for example, children and grandchildren coming to stay as they would have done in the old family home). But they make clear, from their research in Canada, that the ideal is for adaptations and support to come to the home, rather than older people moving out, because ". . . *allowing older residents to remain in their house is a way to maintain home as the locus of socialization*" (pg 336). In the context of a housing shortage, 'bedroom tax', shrinking resources to supported integrated housing, health and social care support, this option in England is increasingly difficult to implement. There are other ways of encouraging inter-generational connection, particularly in purpose-built housing schemes for the elderly. Recent examples from the Netherlands show schemes where younger people live with older people, sometimes in their home, but also in purposefully designed housing schemes. The benefit for older people is the company, the youthful energy and engagement. For the younger generation, the benefits are learning from wisdom and experience and sharing the increasingly burdensome housing costs.

Co-housing is one of the potential answers to our shortage of affordable housing and to increasing reports of isolation and loneliness. It could be inter-generational by design. It might be a response to homelessness and as a step to more sustainable housing. There are many benefits to sharing spaces and places, even where the thought of it is uncomfortable as an abstract concept. There are those reporting the positive benefits of living together, not necessarily in family units, but as we've seen in spaces designed for strangers to connect – sharing our places and our lives.

Conclusion

Feeling 'at home' is inherently emotional. Our identity(ies) are at an inter-section at home as much as they are beyond the threshold. Some of that is related to what goes on within – the people we share our home and our neighbouring spaces with; but some is from outside – insecurity of the space itself.

Planning for, and living in, homes, is an emotional process. Government policy and local authority practice on the supply and delivery of 'homes' (housing) needs to recognise this. Conflict (and the need for negotiation) should be recognised in the process of planning for homes. The antagonistic practices of place and identity connecting – needs to be seen and recognised in laws and policies around the use of home, the need for support to find home and to utilise it well – to feel secure, able to work on our aspirations for happy lives, connected with people and places.

3 Protecting home
Negotiating conflict

Introduction

Emotional attachment to home, and the space around it, is amplified in the moments when we are less certain about the security of place and our accommodation. Precarity of home – for example when threatened with homelessness (rooflessness) creates tension and conflict of place and identity. This chapter starts with conflict within our home – the consideration that home can trap people, or make people feel trapped. Converse to our aims for home – it can deplete our reserves of energy. Home may be the place where social labour is exercised without reward or recognition – caring, cooking, cleaning, in many cases adversely affecting and discriminating against women. In extreme cases it can be a place of imprisonment – modern day slavery in homes, reportedly on the increase. In extreme cases, where domestic and family violence is perpetrated, home is a place where people (again disproportionately women) are bruised, battered and controlled – home can turn into a murder scene.

This chapter will also examine wider planning-process community conflict – disputes between community members on where housing should be built, where people should be able to live; and I offer suggestions on negotiating conflict, reflecting on lessons from some of my research project findings. Conflict within home and with community can lead to a strong urge to protect home and family; this is seen in the popularisation amongst the wealthy elite, to live in gated communities. However, one can ask – are we gating in or out? This desire to protect not just family and home, but notional financial values and enjoyment of property can lead to cognitive dissonance. How can we know objectively of the importance of a home, but also deny others access to home through objection to others being built? It is necessary to mediate conflict of home within four walls, between homes on streets or sites.

Home is messy and complex, place is constantly being redefined as are our own connections with it – our identities. As Doreen Massey reminds us:

"The thrown togetherness of place demands negotiation" (Massey, 2005, pg 141).

Home as a site of social depletion

Home can be a site of depletion, domestic drudgery, unhappiness and sometimes domestic violence. This part of the chapter will examine the range of ways this happens. For example, at one end of the spectrum, there will be many (particularly women still) who will feel exhausted by all the work that home creates; there is an element of gendered social depletion through home 'work' and how that disadvantages, mostly, women. At the other end of the spectrum, there is outright criminal activity taking place behind the privacy of the front door of 'home', such as control, coercion, physical domestic and family violence, as well as imprisonment of vulnerable migrants for domestic and sex work – modern slavery. The numbers for human trafficking and modern slavery have risen in recent years. Whilst left unchecked, the front door can act as the barricade between a caring society and an imprisoned person, it is important that organisations in government, and in the social housing sector, take a lead in tackling modern slavery and domestic violence. There are examples where multi-agency working has failed in protecting children and vulnerable people. From Victoria Climbie, to Baby P to Fiona Pilkington – all in hindsight with many visible flags to social services and other agencies that urgent intervention was necessary – all died following failure to do so.

Many social housing organisations will have social responsibility statements, safeguarding policies, domestic violence procedures, and more recently modern slavery statements (following the Modern Slavery Act, 2015). The numbers of people trapped as modern slaves, behind closed doors, belies the occasional headline of illegal immigrants kept to work for little or nothing by seemingly 'nice' families. The Salvation Army (2017) reported a 300% increase on people referring to their service. Social housing organisations are ostensibly the 'always there' service – not parachuting in for a social or health emergency, but month-by-month collecting the rent, maintaining the property, in contact with their residents enough to notice things when they're wrong – before they escalate. However, there are pressures on the social housing service, which mean such opportunities to notice when things might be wrong, and to intervene, are increasingly designed out through a self-serve approach to service delivery. This impacts on residents and service users, but also on those housing officers working in the social housing sector, trying to provide the support needed to maintain 'home'.

Emotional depletion in the home affects those living in that place, but it also causes vicarious trauma and reduced resilience in the workplace in the agencies and organisations providing social housing and other services to support people make and maintain 'home'. In research for the Chartered Institute of Housing (Richardson et al., 2014) on the future of 'frontline' housing work, one of the findings was the increased level of anxiety and potential depletion of resilience amongst those working in the sector to deal with first and second hand trauma. First-hand trauma was felt because housing workers themselves need a home, and they also face the pressures on affordability of and access to secure housing. Second-hand, or vicarious trauma was really evident in some of the accounts shared by workers in the research (and continues to be shared in conversations today). They reported how they were emotionally affected by hearing from residents who were homeless or facing homelessness, who couldn't afford the rent, who couldn't afford to eat, who couldn't see how to carry on, some who felt the only way out was suicide. This is a space of ongoing research in my work: to continue examining the impact of austerity on residents in (or hoping to access) social housing, the resulting trauma felt in the sector, and the impact on those working on the frontline in delivering housing management and support (and indeed those working in research and education for housing management staff).

Gilroy and Woods (1994) in their edited collection note that women have a particular relationship with home – that there is a gendered dimension. They reported then, that women on their own find it harder to access owner occupation, and remain in that sector post-divorce. In that book, Darke (1994) notes the complex relationship women have with home, which echoes the thoughts of Gilman (1903). Darke notes:

> *there is a distinctive relationship between women and their homes; that women value their homes in a particular way. Our feelings are a mixture of affection, reciprocated towards the home as a nurturing environment, and resentment at the demands of the home.*

(Darke, 1994, pg 11)

We know this complicated relationship with home to be a daily lived experience, to be loved and exhausted by home and to reconstruct ourselves within that space, and in our place in society, day in day out. This goes beyond purely personal costs. Indeed ,Gilman in 1903 looked beyond personal individual costs to women and embraced the more expansive cost of the influence of home on women, men, children, society and the economy. At the thinner end of the wedge of damage that home can do to women, is social reproduction and depletion. Elson (2000) discuss depletion of human capabilities through unpaid work, supporting globalised economies. Rai et al. (2013) clarify that social reproduction for women happens in the space where

> *there is a critical gap between the outflows – domestic, affective and reproductive – and the inflows that sustain their health and well-being.*
>
> (Rai et al., 2013, pg 86)

Over a sustained period, say Rai et al. (2013), this gap between sustaining inflow and reproductive outflow is harmful to those engaged in the unvalued work. They make clear, as well, that the harm is incurred beyond the individual. Three main 'sites of depletion' can be found: at the level of the individual engaged in the unvalued work, at the level of the household, and also at the level of the community. Within these sites, there are multiple ways in which harm can manifest. Rai et al. (2013, pgs 91–92) note four types of harm that can occur as a result of social reproduction:

1   Discursive harm
2   Emotional harm
3   Bodily harm
4   Harm to citizenship entitlements

As constructors and consumers of 'home' we can see this. In the first instance for discursive harm, this is evident through the (non)value placed on domestic activities to create home – still. The value that society (through political and media discourse) places on the important domestic work that goes into home (maintaining place and caring for people) does not reflect the work and emotional labour invested. The emotional harm relates to guilt associated with being at home, or not being at home. Working mothers and non-working mothers feel guilty, alike, for opposite reasons. Being present in the office (with home in the head) is both difficult, but also a guilt-ridden relief from domestic drudgery. Being present in the home (with either the office in the head, or dreams of escaping undervalued drudgery) is also a challenge. This particular issue – being present in the home – is explored a little more in the next chapter (4) in considering whether our performance at home is a private or a public performance. In addition to emotional harm, the third type of harm pointed out by Rai et al. (2013) is bodily harm. They reflect on the (non)regulation of the body of the worker within the home. The work of birth, caring, cleaning can take physical tolls on the body as well as emotional impacts on the mind. Rai et al.'s fourth and final type of harm – to citizenship entitlements – links to emotional value but places this firmly within (non) contribution to the economy. This is structured in to the economy and the state and manifests very clearly. One example is in the pensions of 'baby boomer' women who will have contributed to seemingly valueless (but priceless) work in the home – social reproduction – but because they weren't 'working' and making national insurance contributions through salaried employment, they may have a lower pension to draw on in their old age, unless subsequent credits have been purchased to top-up. Not valued for caring in the home behind closed doors when they were of working age – not recompensed in older age when they need caring for. This leads to harm through (lack of) citizenship entitlements as a result of social reproduction.

Home-trap

Home can be physically dangerous. The place itself can be dangerous to physical and emotional health – damp, poor wiring, noisy. Some places have historical renown for danger. One particular development in nineteenth-century London was depicted by a novelist Arthur Morrison. Boughton (2018) tells us the novel's description of this place, the Old Nichol in London, was only lightly fictionalised and that:

> *The Old Nichol usually killed more insidiously, however, through disease and deprivation. Its death rates were over twice the London average; one in four newborns were likely to die before their first birthday. In 1891, just before its clearance, 5,719 people lived in the district, three-quarters of them in one and two-room dwellings, in houses built with 'billy-sweet' a mortar including street dirt which never dried out. That, as well as fetid humanity, would explain the characteristic aroma which Morrison identified.*

(Boughton, 2018, pgs 9–10)

Whilst places like the Old Nichol no longer exist, and there have been rounds of slum clearances from cities in the UK since then, ostensibly to improve lives (but also gentrifying and increasing values for land and property owners too), there are still modern day places which are dangerous, cramped – hiding physical and emotional harm behind closed doors.

Even when, from the outside, there may have been physical refurbishment, the improved veneer itself can become a death-trap, as was seen in the tragedy of Grenfell Tower. This is where 'housing as home' is an important political and philosophical space. Home, indeed, is a social construction created and recreated by the people who live in or near. But it is also, in the context of house as home, a physical construct which needs regulating for safety and security. Government's place in home, is in this space of regulating housing as home; its role is to protect those who trust and are complacent about the safety of a place managed by government agencies, or registered social landlords. The increasing march of housing as home into the private rented sphere (at the cost of social rented housing) makes the link for government regulation of safe home, more tenuous. Government should not allow capitalist market ideas of profit and physical value of housing run free in the space of housing as home – there is a role for political leadership and regulation to ensure the physical safety of home.

In addition to the housing, the physical construction itself, being a danger, there are many cases where it is the social construction – the people within home – who also present a trap. This is most notably seen in the figures and the debate around domestic and family violence.

Internationally, 95% of perpetrators of homicide are male and two-thirds of victims are women. Thirty per cent of women who have had an intimate relationship have suffered violence from their intimate partner. Half of the violent crimes against women in England and Wales in 2015 were domestic abuse related (Walby et al., 2017) Domestic violence is devastating; it is gendered and it can be hidden behind closed doors in a world where 'an English man's home is his (private) castle'. Walby et al. (2017) highlight the devastation of such violence:

> *Violence matters. It wrecks lives. It causes injury and misery. Violence is both a cause and consequence of inequality. It is a violation of human rights. Violence is a detriment to health and to sustainable economic development.*
>
> (Walby et al., 2017, pg 1)

The Domestic Abuse Housing Alliance (DAHA) is an example of the passion for protecting 'home' held by social housing leaders and charities. Founded by two housing associations and a charity – Gentoo, Standing Together, and Peabody – in 2014, they have raised the profile of this issue in the social housing sector significantly, to the point where domestic violence was the key theme and charitable aim of the Chartered Institute President in 2017. DAHA is an important campaign, framing improved approaches in the sector through accreditation of organisations, policies and procedures – to help drawback the secrecy and stigma, to raise the profile of the issue and to support social housing providers to involve themselves in cases where intervention and support is needed.

Shenai et al. (2018) in their research for DAHA founding member Gentoo, offered a range of practical and policy recommendations for housing providers to be involved in solutions for domestic violence. One such recommendation was to increase the profile and understanding of this issue with staff and tenants. Housing is an 'always there' service – observing daily life, able to pick up on changes in circumstance, more than the emergency 'parachute' services like emergency health, police and social services. If domestic violence is raised as an issue, through publicity campaigns and training, then staff and neighbours are better placed to help. Early detection and support was also identified as key, using information for example on repairs calls, to identify where an issue might be domestic violence related. Working with agencies in collaboration was noted, as with many social problems, as vital to successful intervention. The research also recommended that perpetrator behaviour was targeted, for example by structuring domestic violence into the tenancy agreement, making removal of the perpetrator from the home simpler to achieve, through noncompliance with the tenancy agreement. This puts the onus on the perpetrator, rather than the victim, something that is seen in practice in some locations, where there are examples of the victim being enabled to remain in the family home, to stay safe with support, having removed the perpetrator.

Spinney (2012) reports on her research for AHURI, examining domestic and family violence in Australia and in England, that a mix of approaches is vital – intertwining legal, housing and welfare approaches to the support that is necessary. She notes the growing orthodoxy of understanding that women and children should not be made homeless as a response to them being a victim of domestic violence crime, and there are examples of sanctuary approaches in England and in Australia in the report. We need to move more quickly into a new way of doing things. This would involve housing organisations stepping more proactively into the space, to lead on the coordinated response to keep women safe in their own home; and it can be seen in networks like the Domestic Abuse Housing Alliance in England, to create a space for developing this further.

Domestic violence puts women and children at risk of physical and emotional harm. One tenet of the abuse is isolation, through tactics of coercion and control. Warrington (2001) notes:

> *This isolation from normal social contact and the unreality of being frequently subjected to abuse, make it very difficult for women to know where to turn. Thus leaving home is invariably the outcome of many years of abuse, sometimes characterized by several episodes of leaving and returning.*

(pgs 372–373)

Women can feel trapped, either in the home because they are controlled by a partner, or in a refuge if it is away from wider social networks and support. As part of recovery, the sufferers of domestic violence need to talk with people who have had similar experiences and who may understand, but they also need to build resilience through both bonding and bridging capital (Putnam, 2010) – through being able to step outside the door and rebuild networks.

> *The spatial patterns of women's perceptions of risk, of the actual risks they are exposed to, and of their behavioural responses have implications for their equal participation in society.*

(Pain, 1991, pg 415)

This point on gendered spatial inequality resulting from violence or fear of violence, is problematic when it is hidden behind 'privacy of home'. The higher rates of violence against women, the numbers of women controlled and coerced in the home means that the private space within which such crime is perpetrated needs to have porous walls – where 'home' can be allowed to breathe in through the spaces created by social, housing, crime and health policy which mean women must not be allowed to suffer, isolated and alone.

Dryden (1999) reminds us of the gendered power imbalance of marriage, which holds a mirror up to power in the home.

> *Statistically, women are much more at risk of being attacked, raped or murdered in their own home by their husband or male partner than they are of being attacked, raped or murdered by a stranger. (It was only in 1991 that a law was passed in this country making rape in marriage illegal).*

(Dryden, 1999, pg 10)

Organisations, like Peabody, who recognise and face the issue of domestic violence, and who lead the sector in responding to it, may initially see reporting of domestic violence increase, as victims are supported and encouraged to disclose what might previously have remained suspected but ultimately hidden. The action, as noted by Spinney (2012) is not solely for housing, but should be related to legal and welfare responses, too. Additionally, the response from multiple agencies and from wider societal breaking of taboos, should be for the long term, years after the bruises have healed. We know that domestic violence is a predominant factor amongst the causes of homelessness. It should also be recognised that the effects of domestic violence on sustainable housing responses are long term. O'Campo et al. (2016) discussed 'psychological instability' of housing for domestic violence survivors that must be recognised over time, in addition to the physical instability of housing around a specific violent episode. The preferable option, through a housing, legal and welfare network of support would be to evict the perpetrator and to keep women and children safe in their own home. The longer term psychological housing stability would flourish more, where the victim had not been made homeless as a result of the crime. Where a victim did have to leave their home for safety, Sullivan and Olsen (2016) note that a 'housing first' type approach to homelessness shares many traits with domestic violence advocacy, including, increasingly, trauma-informed practice.

Conflict in planning for home

The emotional collateral tied up in home creates complex responses when things threaten to change around the home: for example, a new housing development, a waste disposal plant or other unwanted land use. There are various shades of unknown and unwanted in the types of new development and some objections are based on fears of impact on health, others on house values for example. The prospect of change in the neighbourhood initiates a reflection on the meaning of our home to us.

If we think about the complexity of the response in objection to planning applications for new developments there are tangible issues, such as house values, impact on health, which can be measured and monitored, and there are further underlying reasons that are less tangible, such as fear of the 'other' (Richardson, 2006).

In King's (2010) discussion of home, there is a strong link with individual households protected by the walls that enclose them. In his social constructionist approach in the development of the idea of 'housing pathway' Clapham (2002) problematises the term 'household' and highlights that it is important to look outside of just one 'unit':

Interaction with neighbours and others in the wider geographical area will also be an important element of the consumption of the house. This may tie in to the presence or absence of a sense of community which may be manifest in interaction with neighbours or to the esteem in which the area is held and in the attitudes towards the area held by outsiders or the press. This may also be an important factor in identity and lifestyle.

(pg 64)

In contentious planning decisions, those individual walls can break down and the 'us' becomes wider; it can include the street, neighbourhood or community. In the case of local people protecting against the 'unwanted', collectives are built where they may previously have not existed.

Madanipour talks about planning today being a formal framework, underneath which is a more informal system of networks making connections.

The connections that have to be made, he says, '*can be functional, causal, formal, temporal or spatial*' (pg 363) but that '*These connections, therefore, may be contingent rather than consolidated, and simplifying rather than responding to diversity and complexity*' (pg 366).

Different aspects of space are the source for conflict in the planning system on many planning applications whether for new homes, or other contentious developments such as wind farms or waste disposal plants. Conflict and contradiction in perception of space can create huge tension in individual planning applications for unwanted but necessary services, or in applications to develop a larger quantity of homes. However, Innes and Booher (2010) suggest that contradiction in and of itself should not necessarily be avoided:

> *The world is in constant motion, and everything we admire has a dark side, which may emerge at any time. The yin and yang of collaboration cannot be avoided so it must be embraced. Agonism can be creative, spurring us to address dilemmas and problems, and keeping us from complacency.*
>
> (pgs 112–113)

Porter's (2010) research focused on colonial cultures of planning and its impact on the Indigenous people of Australia, finding that oppression and colonial history and dominance were ever present. Reflecting on her position of speaking 'from' (as a planner) and 'to' (as a researcher) planning as a profession in Australia, she wondered about the voice of planning:

> *If planning is a producer of place, what does it claim is worth producing and how is this particular view of the world continually mediated and reconstituted?*
>
> (pg 16)

There are parallels to be drawn between the seemingly increasingly tightening regulatory approach to planning for Gypsies and Travellers in England and for Indigenous Aboriginal people in Australia – geographically marginalised historically through reservations. Formalisation of use of space, focused policing and tight control over access to common places in England has created fewer and fewer traditional places for Gypsies and Travellers to live. Informal and meanwhile use of land for traditional communities has been formally planned out of modern use of space.

The perception of space itself is also an emotional consideration; the earlier discussion of Lefebvre's work showed that the connection between human beings and space prohibited a purely abstract view of planning space, because it is lived experience. So, as important as it is to consider reasoning and objective criteria, as noted by Fisher and Ury (1999), it is also necessary to consider emotions such as fear, in the debate on planning for sites. Baum (2011) suggests that: *"Planning and policy analysis give little attention to how societal institutions and culture influence the expression of largely unconscious desires and anxieties in ways that create social inequality and shape policies that do little to reduce it"* (pg 103). A psychoanalytical approach to the issues and identities wrapped up on planning places, can improve understanding in this area. This is echoed by Gunder (2011) who suggests that planning is not just a practical function but instead has an *"ideologically shaping role in the formulation of our desires for our future communities"* (pg 325). Porter (2010) in her conclusion on unlearning colonial planning practices in relation to the Indigenous people in Australia, refers to the work of bell hooks (1994) on love; she makes clear that in planning terms this is not an over-sentimentalised theory, but a practice:

> *Instead, it is love as a deep practice of connection: of selflessness, humility and compassion. It is not a 'model' of being or a set of rules, but an ethic towards others, a daily practice.*
>
> (Porter, 2010, pg 157)

Emotion is increasingly prominent in the business world. It is also there in government in the application of behavioural economics, or 'nudge', in attempts to shape citizen responses to issues (Richardson, 2010). Hill (2008) suggests that *'emotion drives reason more than reason drives emotion'* (pg 17) and that feelings are a filter for information processing. Fear and contradiction – strong feelings – can facilitate action and unearth entrenched power imbalances. This might not necessarily result in more homes, the action created by fear could be in campaigning to stop a particular development or 'protecting' through gating out.

Gates of fear and anti-social spaces

Minton (2009) draws on an analogy of a picture in her analysis of gated communities:

> *making me think how gates frame places, picking out the space and highlighting it. While a frame is an appropriate way of drawing attention to a picture, places are not gallery spaces, and gates, like frames, make the space outside the gates seem less important . . .*
>
> (pg 69)

Gates, and other physical partitions, create fragmented spaces – whether the gates frame a more or less important section of society, they are marked out as other. Gates can keep people out, or trap people in (the latter example being seen in the iconic scaffolding which acted as a gate to the Travellers site at Dale Farm, keeping police and bailiffs out).

Graham (2011) suggests that there is increasing militarisation of urban spaces. We can see this in how we talk about space, plan and govern space, and indeed how we live, work and play in urban spaces. Militarisation, and the use of military language in urban planning, is normalised. It also relies on an 'us' and a 'them' and 'our' and 'their' links with space, based on their and our social construction of identity and place.

Space that wasn't felt to be owned (and defended) could become a place that, rather than everyone taking responsibility and pleasure from it, indeed no one did, and it became an empty space to be filled with crime, anti-social space. The premise was then that space needed to be 'owned' – defended – the term defensible space (Newman, 1972) already sounding more like a war zone than a home zone. Wilson and Kelling (1982) in their theory on 'Broken Windows' talked of the different perception of space and of the role of the police in managing space, between smaller towns and big urban cities. They noted that in the smaller towns and cities, there was perhaps more *'sensitivity to communal as opposed to individual needs'* (pg 36). A communal approach to land and place means that it is everyone's rather than no-one's and so there is contribution to the daily lived experience, rather than 'defence' that is required. Coleman (1990) also relates to the architecture of the designed space in her book *Utopia on Trial*, which looked at communal areas in high-rise blocks and the anti-social behaviour and crime that occurred in these undefended and un-owned spaces. Modern architecture in the city has created potential for the creation of home and work spaces for many, but it has also caused offence to some – Wolfe (1982) was scathing in his reflection on the limitations of utopia in American modern architecture. But, of course, we are reminded by Jane Jacobs (1961), in her ground-breaking work: safety in the city is not delivered best through architectural devices, or through technology – but rather through people, their senses – their eyes and ears seeing what was happening on the sidewalks: knowing their neighbours:

> *The first thing to understand is that the public peace – the sidewalk and street peace – of cities is not kept primarily by the police, necessary as police are. It is kept primarily by an intricate, almost unconscious, network of voluntary controls and standards among the people themselves, and enforced by the people themselves.*

> (Jacobs, 1961, pg 40)

Contrary to this people-centred approach to safety and security – humans on the street keeping an eye out – there is a growing phenomenon of physical security responses, to keep danger out. Atkinson and Blandy (2017) show a range of illustrated examples of gating across the globe – many of these serve to illustrate their point that 'gating begets gating':

> *What some see as the apparent social disorder lying outside protected residential zones, itself produced by forms of social disinvestment and welfare retrenchment, have helped to legitimise the ways the affluent have divided themselves from more deprived groups through gating, guarding and 'forting-up', and the rise of aggressive responses to poverty by states and citizens. Gating begets gating, so the fortress home percolates through the urban fabric and generates hostility between class positions.*

(Atkinson and Blandy, 2017, pg 160)

Increasingly, cities are segregated and regimented, and they can feel 'closed' Sennett (2018). This is a growing phenomenon in the way cities are designed, built, policed and experienced on a daily basis – and it is spreading from the global North to the South. Sennett (2018) argues that we need more 'open' cities for resident wellbeing, and that a level of planning experimentation is required. What is referred to as 'fortressing-up' by Atkinson and Blandy (2017) links to the notion of an Englishman's home as 'his castle'; and they remind us of the origin of this saying in law is to protect homeowners from the intrusion of the state. They discuss this concept (pg 142) in relation to the law in the U.S.A where the links between popular film culture and the imagination of home as castle have created the 'Castle Doctrine', 'Make My Day' and 'Stand your Ground' legislation in the U.S.A. The use of maximum force to defend home (remember that with its inextricable link with identity, it is difficult to delineate 'home' and 'us': intrusion into home is intrusion into us). This is so much a taken-for-granted approach that the many killings in this zone are categorised as 'justifiable homicides' and not recorded in any detail. In the U.K there is less of an appetite for this 'maximum force' approach, but there are cases where justifiable force can be used in defence of home. In April 2018, in a case which must have ticked many news editors' boxes, a Gypsy man was killed by a home owner in South London during an alleged burglary. The police and crime prosecution service concluded that on the basis of the evidence, there would be no further action against the home-owner. Relatives of the deceased tried to leave flowers and notes as a shrine, outside the place where he was killed (the home of the man who killed him in self-defence) but these were torn down several times. This very complex legal and social event, unfortunately, got turned into an 'us and them' classical tabloid tale of Gypsies intruding and homeowners defending. This simplistic media portrayal of an intricate issue is not new – one more example of Gypsies and Travellers used as signals to 'us' to other 'them'; rather than a news piece about two men allegedly attempting to undertake a home burglary, one of whom was killed by the owner defending the property. The Gypsy ethnic status of the burglar, a red-herring, used to simplify the tale and sell the news.

One important part of the physical apparatus of securitised cities – gated communities – is the surveillance equipment, which exerts control over the activity within a space. The CCTV camera is a physical manifestation of the 'gaze' of power.

> *the gaze is not faithful to truth, nor subject to it, without asserting, at the same time, a supreme mastery: the gaze that sees is a gaze that dominates.*

> (Foucault, 1969, pg 39)

In this work by Foucault, which explored the way doctors looked at illnesses in their patients, the power of the gaze was not just in the observation, but in the interpretive element. In a city, one person's hooded criminal loitering with intent, is another's beloved teenage son spending time with his friends – boisterous not bad. The interpretative perception of the observer is a controlling element of 'gaze'. Mix this scope for (mis)interpretation of people and behaviour, with the planned use of space as just one element of the 'lived reality' of place (Lefebvre, 1991) and it is easy to see how different dreams of the use of space can clash. What behaviour should happen in a space? Is it the case that youth shouldn't be able to crowd together in communal or public places? Physical design, signs asking people not to gather, drink, play ball games, even high pitched noise used to cause discomfort to teenage ears more than adults, are part of the controlling apparatus of urban space – to 'defend' it.

The very presence of a CCTV camera (whether or not it is recording) the perception of being observed and (mis)interpreted, has an effect on our behaviour. This phenomenon of the thought of being observed was noted by Foucault (1977) in his thoughts on Bentham's Panopticon design for the prison. If people are potential targets of structured societal gaze, then they begin to internalise the gaze and become their own police – controlling actions in anticipation that they may or may not be observed. With the plethora of surveillance cameras capturing the detailed movement in urban spaces, the march of the securitisation, the militarisation of the city becomes ever faster, ever invasive in the name of 'defence' of spaces.

This is not to decry surveillance equipment as deterrent altogether – I have seen people plead for reinstatement of CCTV cameras outside their site to try to prevent those who had threatened to take it over from actually doing so. There is a clear benefit to deterring crime, and to catching criminals where there are a lot of people sharing a small geographical area. CCTV can help catch crime hidden behind closed doors, it can reassure. The challenge comes when amplified security and surveillance changes the nature of people and places, alters and control behaviours that may not be criminal (just perhaps contradictory and not universally enjoyed across generations). Civic measures to police space, such as injunctions related to use of common land in a town or city, when broken can result in a criminal offence and punishment. What may start as 'defence' measures to create better shared spaces, can turn into the criminalisation of different behaviours, alternative uses and claims on common land and spaces. One person's bench is another's skate-boarding stunt; one person's dog walking park may be another's annual stopping place, used by the family for centuries. We should be utilising design, planning, policy and practice to allow a diversity of uses – negotiated by communities – rather than a hegemonic approach to a monochrome method of controlling place.

The term 'social' and 'anti-social' have changed in housing discourse and practice. As a housing practitioner starting out managing my 'patch' in the 1990's, I dealt with something called 'neighbour nuisance'. This was before 'anti-social behaviour' was common parlance in social housing management or legislation. Neighbour nuisance required visits with enough time for a chat over tea and biscuits, negotiation with both or more parties, resulting in written letters recording the agreed course of action. Where the disagreement was about more than playing ball games in an area where a sign said 'no ball games' or, in one case: disagreement about the acceptable number of garden gnomes in a space, then this was escalated. Sometimes this was because the alleged action was anti-social to the wider community; often the behaviour was evidently in breach of tenancy conditions and was acted on accordingly. Today, the term neighbour nuisance is rarely used, it falls within the wider term of 'anti-social behaviour' (ASB). There are a range of tools that can be used by housing organisations to deter and to deal with ASB, but this is another area where the initial intervention is through civil law, but the remedy, if the initial order is broken, becomes a criminal matter.

Negotiating conflict

Fragmented societies create challenges for planning (Healey, 2006) and there is a need to recognise difference, understand past trauma and engage in participatory planning processes so that communities get to know each other better (Forester, 1999, 2009). Space is contested and it is represented and perceived in different ways. Forester (2009) suggests that ". . . *as we differ on basic beliefs . . . we might still come to agree upon specific practical actions . . .*" (pg 91). Healey (2006) adds that through mediation and discursive practices people come to understand different points of view, reflect on their own view, and that ". . . *a store of mutual understanding is built up . . .*" (pg 33). Kaufman and Smith (1999) propose that conflict over land use issues are framed and reframed as part of the reconciliation of differences (pg 165).

Decision-making in planning cases can be messy, complex and the source of conflict. Indeed Mintzberg and Westley (2001) conclude that a rational approach of: define, diagnose, design and decide is an uncommon process (pg 89). Instead, they suggest decisions are made beyond the limits of 'think first' and are in fact supplemented with 'see first' and 'do first' models (pg 89). Hudson and Lowe (2009) discuss decision-making that goes beyond rational choice explanations to include human agency and chaos in the mix. Parsons (1995) probes the differences between decision-making approaches, summarising that:

> *Managerialism (especially when allied to 'public choice' theory) in this sense represents an on-going search to take decision-making out of a world where there are conflicts over values and beliefs into a realm where decisions can be made in a more rational (non-political) way.*
>
> (Parsons, 1995, pg 454)

Purely rational, non-political decision-making is not possible in planning for housing either on a strategic plan-making level or on individual criteria-based decisions for individual planning applications or appeals. The issues involved are so inherently value-laden that rationality is constrained. As Forester (1999) reminds us: "*Decision making involves not only cognitive choice but social expression . . .*" (pg 150).

Laws and Forester (2015) suggest conflict as the stage for improvisation; and in earlier work Forester (2009) talked of not mystifying value differences, ". . . *even in the face of deep value differences, many practical resolutions may be possible, even if – or indeed because – asking parties to change their fundamental beliefs is often neither necessary nor relevant to settling the dispute at hand*" (pg 79). Indeed in research for the Joseph Rowntree Foundation (Richardson, 2007) it was found that practical cases could be made to gain political support for accommodation delivery through economic and legal arguments, rather than moral/social (more value-laden) arguments – separation of positions and interests was key to negotiation.

For new development, it is also the case that places and spaces can be imbued with different values. Lefebvre's (1991) triad of perceived space, conceived space and lived space can help to conceptualise these changing values. Housing development proposals, particularly on areas of land designated as 'green belt' in the countryside, include the placing of values on people, as well as the social construction of perceived space (representations of space). This requires participants in a negotiation on sites to step back from getting entrenched in values on two levels; people and place. Al Ramiah and Hewstone (2013) write on the possibility of 'contact theory' as a tool to resolve differences between groups; and in their evaluation of a school project in the North of England where entrenched perceived differences between ethnic groups were held, children started to find common ground after being put together in the classroom. But, within the topic of planning for accommodation of different types for a range of individuals and communities, there is also a need for better understanding of different people's perception of the land in question and a sharing of the cultural history of a place, to better understand the origin of different parties' proposals or objections.

Susan Podziba in her (2012) book *Civic Fusion* refers to a reaction to inertia – a realisation that the status quo benefits no-one, as one of the essential conditions for civic fusion. The heads are still in the sand on a number of accommodation projects in many areas – local authorities haven't yet reached 'peak inertia' in order to galvanise action (particularly for non-standard housing for marginalised groups); but in others there has been a moment, perhaps a point of conflict that has galvanised action towards resolution and better accommodation management and delivery.

Sanyal (2005, pg 236) suggests that planners must learn how to better formulate problems:

> *Problems must be formulated not on the basis of what planners know about their complexity, but on the simplest ways that something can be done about them. This would make problem formulation an exercise in which planners anticipate the types of resistance their policies are likely to evoke from both inside and outside the state, and strategize how such resistance can be minimized, bypassed, or best turned into supporting forces.*

Some key steps for strategic planners who wish to see housing, particularly social housing or 'non-traditional' housing actualised, should include: (1) anticipate resistance, include methods of negotiation in conceptualising the plan (2) coalition building inside and outside the bureaucratic network, (3) facilitation of spaces and frameworks for opposing groups to negotiate,

(4) understand planning and implementation are not separate activities, but part of the same continuum and (5) leaders in local government must take seriously their role to plan accommodation for disadvantaged and marginalised groups.

Conclusions

This chapter has attempted to throw the light and shade of home into a framework of planning and negotiation. Home is security and love, but is also conflict and control. It is a private space to be our authentic selves – a platform from which to perform. But it can also be a home-trap, a place of violence and fright. Sometimes home is a prison – a place where a partner controls, but it might also be a place where we gate ourselves in. Moreover, the gating can be contagious, damaging the wider social fabric – making us consider that space outside: is it everyone's or no-one's?

As we've seen throughout the book so far, the defining concepts of understanding home – place and identity – are ever moving constructs. As Massey (2005) confides – place is messy, it needs negotiation. Our conflicting notions of identity and our links with geographical space create a need to constantly re-negotiate place – if we are all to find our 'home' in a connected way, rather than from behind gates.

4 Home screen
A public or private performance?

Introduction

The onset of new technology creates a 'home screen' that is not necessarily one that protects us. Indeed, it may 'protect' (preclude) us from authentic human connection with people inside our four walls. Virtual conversations online connecting us outside, but when the device is switched off (if it ever is) loneliness can pervade the physical space. Our 'home screen' could hide our real self, whilst amplifying (inauthentic) images of 'home'. This chapter asks, in the age of Facebook, how private is home – and does this matter for our understanding of what home is and what purpose it serves?

The home has traditionally been a site of collective activity – eating together at the kitchen table, watching television programmes in front of the family TV set. Modern technology allows entertainment to be on demand, bespoke to what we want and when we want it. Streaming services and multiple (endless) channels require numerous TV sets, smart phones and tablet devices. Once, the household may have consumed TV (and meals) together, but modern schedules see individuals in different parts of the house, undertaking individual activity. Are we home together but alone? Perhaps, instead, so-called 'social media' which can be consumed virtually, and physically alone, creates unsocial homes and communities.

Online worlds

Shaw and Shaw (2015) explore the laws of cyber communities and online worlds:

> *While the idea of a world directed by human laws and made great by human initiative, endeavour, and passion has to some extent been super-seded, the idealised cyber-community is often purported to assume an antagonistic relationship with the real. The difference between human-*

directed principles and physically-bounded laws of nature versus the unlimited temporal and spatial possibilities of the internet presents a range of seemingly impossible dualisms: intuition and rationality, sensation and ideas, body and machine.

(pg 5)

The intersection between the online world and the real world, at home, is complicated. We can be at home, but not present at home. The distraction of the online world can call to us, let us be somewhere else in the world from the convenience of our own sitting room. Television opened up this world decades ago – who needed to go to the actual game, when you could see the sporting action more close-up on the TV screen? Why explore a potentially hazardous, humid jungle, when instead we can let Attenborough narrate scenes we couldn't possibly expect to actually see if we went ourselves, whilst we have a cup of tea and a biscuit, in our armchair? The answer of course is connection, with other beings. To taste the pint of Guinness and Balti pie at Welford Road and discuss with friends how we of course would have thrown a rugby ball with more precision in a line-out. To hear the sounds and smell the scents of those far-flung places in the globe, along with the anticipation, of maybe, if I hold really still, seeing, hearing, smelling, being in the vicinity of a particular animal in a wild place.

However, the world has moved on, and the social media world provides even more interaction and connection than television – indeed, it is so immersive, it can be addictive. It might not yet provide the full experience of pie and pint with the frustrated expert spectator; but it allows for real-time conversation, sharing of images and ideas. It provides a channel of communication for people who cannot leave their home, through disability perhaps, or through not being able to afford transport and tickets – and it enriches the third-hand experience, making it seem much more real. It can virtually connect us with hundreds, thousands, millions of people watching the same game or protesting the same point. But in connecting through our home screen, beyond home, there is a disconnection with the people in the room with us. We cannot be in two places at once – not in an authentically present way. "I'm just checking my email", or "Let me have five more minutes browsing my snapchats", actually translates to "I am physically here, but mentally absent at home".

Moreover, standing in our kitchen virtually checking out the superior baking skills of a friend can put the existing home space and the resident – us – in a comparatively inferior place. Constant comparison of the performance of home and identity, amongst the domestic goddesses on our Facebook friends list, can create spaces of performance anxiety in our own domain. And yet, in a rational place, we know social media is a performance. Relatively few failed cakes, messy kitchen, dog-sick-on-the-carpet moments make it to a status update. We know this and yet in the social media performance of home and identity, we take other successes at face value, whilst undermining our own.

However, sometimes those moments of failure (when we find them funny, or are feeling isolated and desperate enough to share) do make it online. It is in those virtual sisterhood spaces that (real) parenting tips can be shared, those 'we hear you' moments about non-sleeping children, retired parents needing more time, partners late home from the office (because they can escape the dog-sick noisy messiness of domestic drudgery) can be laughed about and valued by those that know.

The online social media world is our juxtaposed friend and tormentor. Rai et al. (2013) talked about emotional harm as one of four types emerging from social reproduction and depletion. In considering our 'home screen' as home, this can bring emotional support and advice, but also judgement. Other friends' posts online can serve to devalue our own social reproduction emotionally, just as the structure of welfare can devalue domestic work in the home in an economic way. But it can also offer glimpses of sharing stories of failure and drudgery in the domestic sphere which can be cathartic and supportive too.

Social media as a space for connection is a powerful supplement for real-world connection with places, people, sights, smells and touches. But other people's experiences can devalue our own efforts, disproportion can take hold without context and clarification. It can also become a space to mask lived reality. In spinning our domestic performance at home, the drudgery and depletion is hidden behind the screen – amplifying the isolation and loneliness.

Within the physical security and privacy of our four walls, online worlds can be a space for dangers to invade. Extremely private acts can become broadcast to millions. Whitworth (2018) reported on the rise of 'sexploitation' in recent times with people – young men particularly – bribed after being duped into sharing an intimate act online. Thinking they were connected to another young person, anonymous though behind their own home screen, when in fact being part of a purposeful trap by a gang using the images to extort money in return for not publishing them online – too embarrassed to tell family members, people who love them who may be just in the next room, about their embarrassing situation, young people feeling trapped and isolated in their home screen.

Online worlds are also impacting on the physical health and safety of young people in their own homes. Sigman (2017) examined screen dependency disorders in children who spent a lot of 'discretionary' (non-homework) time on a screen – gaming, watching TV. There are neurological concerns around screen addiction, which whilst not necessarily causing dysfunctional affects, recognise the bidirectional relationship between certain behaviours and screen addiction. The all-pervading, immersive presence of online worlds in our homes is making our children more sedentary, fatter – unhealthier, addicted, anxious and depressed.

The home screen is a place where we can literally expose our most private moments, where we can gawp at others, be gawped at, where we can indulge in the most violent immersive games – affecting our neurological responses, but while sitting on our backsides. The home screen can be a place of liberation and connection, but it can also be a danger; and we should apply caution and critique rather than acceptance of inevitable online modernity.

Channel shift

The move to online worlds doesn't just affect individual performances of home. In the realm of increasing efficiencies in public sector services, there are fewer opportunities for human interaction in the processes involved in advising on, letting and management of social housing. This channel shift to online self-services has a disproportionate effect on tenants in an increasingly residualised sector, where the need for support has increased at the same time as austerity policies have reduced support services across the public sector. When loneliness is on the increase, opportunities for real human interaction are decreasing. Whilst there are some examples of housing organisations reducing the size of 'patches' for housing officers and introducing 'coaching' approaches to allow staff to spend the time necessary with tenants who need it – this is not mainstream.

Tenants (as well as those trying to access social housing) are expected to apply for housing online, to pay rents online, to report repairs online. The service that is 'always there', the organisations who are the domestic everyday eyes and ears, able to knit together pieces and bring in support to respond to, for example, a case of domestic violence which might otherwise go unnoticed, is increasingly interacting with many tenants virtually. This leads to the potential of domestic violence, child abuse or domestic slavery cases going undetected because of the lack of physical presence.

In an era of reluctant governance and withdrawal of the state, the job of those working on the frontline in the social housing sector is even more stressful. The external pressures of austerity and welfare reform are manifest in the increasing use of foodbanks as an indicator of poverty; but there are also examples, as found in the *Frontline Futures* research reports from housing officers, of suicide threats from tenants in the face of mounting arrears and benefits sanctions. Regardless of whether a social housing provider has decided to 'reshape its offer' and provide only core services – for those employed in the sector there is a tension between social and commercial, a schism in the values many came into the sector to live up to. There is a felt-responsibility to help those in need.

Dissonance occurs where the felt-responsibility of housing officers is in conflict with the stated new aims of their employer. Where reduction in resources to deliver the service means there is less official time to provide support – amplified somehow through the online disconnection; but individual staff still feel the need to do their best. Council and housing association officers are trying to stretch themselves to continue to support residents who they care about; but this is in danger of becoming almost 'apologetic caring' – stealth support in a wider framework of service reduction.

The Kafkaesque nightmare of the street-level bureaucracy that Daniel Blake faces in the eponymous film by Ken Loach in 2016 is exacerbated by an impossible nexus of 'digital by default' meets 'computer says no'. Absurdly and bleakly funny at the start of the film – it is deadly by the end. In all the talk of public organisations rationalising services, 'channelshifting' communications and access to services online – the humanity of providing care and support is lost. Humanity requires people – real people to provide help and support. The channel shift in housing, and other public services can further isolate people who need human-faced support to prevent them feeling more and more alone.

The commitment, of those working in the social housing sector, to key values of caring and support is remarkable. It is observable just how tiring this emotional input to continue to provide a good service in times of austerity is, and how important 'resilience' is to cope. But leaders and managers in housing organisations must support and nurture the development of resilience, create spaces to share feelings and ideas and attempt to embed this in organisational culture.

Lack of physical connection with people to create places and identities can be isolating for tenants, who have fewer opportunities to connect across public services with human beings who can support them or just listen and be there. Vicarious trauma can be experienced by staff working in housing who may also be living in the sector or who may be in a precarious housing situation themselves in the private rented sector. They hear from tenants who are struggling to pay the rent, but they don't always hear in person, these disembodied conversations can happen through a headset and a 'home screen', in a contact centre, within a framework of targets for number of calls responded to within an hour. Such a framework for communication might not come unstuck when taking a call to repair a tap, but when this is sandwiched with calls of threats to commit suicide, quiet voices explaining that they can't afford to eat or pay the rent – this causes vicarious trauma to the listening member of staff. There is a need for recognition of trauma and resilience in the processes of social housing organisations, so that resilience isn't expected in an internalised 'man-up' sense – but within a context of recognising emotions and providing the spaces in processes to deal with that – as an organisation, as a society.

Privacy

One of the themes in 'home' which emerges from the literature is around space for self – namely privacy. Privacy from the outside world, but also privacy from one another within a dwelling space. King (2004) makes us reflect when he asks: "*But what is the precise nature of privacy? How should we approach it?*" (pg 39). The full range of literature and ideas on 'privacy' cannot be fully analysed within this text, but it has emerged as an important element in some of the reviews on the meaning of home, and in some of the responses in my research projects on homelessness and housing. Privacy is important in the physical security of home, plus in the online home screen, to protect us and our identities.

Going beyond online worlds; the notion of privacy was one of the exploratory lenses used to understand and evaluate an innovative project called '*Freedom 2 Work*' which was responding to homelessness and unemployment in Surrey. In the first two years of the evaluation (2017 and 2018), I spoke to a number of clients about the housing and support offered in the project. One of the issues was around lack of privacy in shared accommodation. Some of the respondents said that sharing accommodation as a young adult was alright, but in mature adulthood it was more awkward, for example in sharing bathroom and kitchen facilities. There is a balance to strike though, with privacy and security on the one hand – isolation and loneliness on the other. Some respondents interviewed noted this, and once the awkwardness of sharing with others had faded, there was potential for connectedness and peer support. One older, male respondent said: "*I suffer from depression and anxiety so it [sharing] was a big thing. I was very worried about moving in with people I didn't know . . . I moved in, the guys were really welcoming, I've made a really good friend there, I'm glad it happened. They say everything happens for a reason – doing a share, it was meant to be, because I made a good friend*".

Privacy is clearly a key element of feeling 'at home' – the ability to shut out the world and feel sheltered from outside pressures. However, privacy brings with it hidden issues in the home, such as domestic violence and exploitation online. It should also be looked at within a wider discussion linked to loneliness too.

Lonely

To be lonely is to be homesick, even sometimes when we're in our house – loneliness can create a feeling that we're not 'at home'. Very many people feel lonely: *"Loneliness, I began to realise, was a populated place: a city in itself"* (Laing, 2017, pg 8).

We can feel lonely even when surrounded by others. Sometimes being with people who do not share our values can make us feel lonelier than if we were alone. Franklin (2009) refers to the 'considerable suffering and pain' of loneliness. Indeed, loneliness is seen increasingly as part of a medical model – a symptom of depressive illness, rather than an outcome of increased 'virtualisation' of social worlds and isolation of securitised urban communities and gated spaces. Social prescriptions are handed out by general practitioners, prescribing people to join a club, or to go out and walk a dog. On the one hand, this is de-chemicalising prescriptions for depression, but on the other hand it is medicalising social connection and exercise. It is bringing social connection within the medical sphere, as something to prescribe to individuals. Reducing dependency on emotional painkillers must be a 'good thing', but this prescription and medicalisation of social connection needs to be more critically reflected upon.

Laing (2017) talks of loneliness as a place, a city, itself; she haunts us with her very personal portrayal of living in New York. Many people live in loneliness – it is a space inhabited by millions. It is not only in New York or London, it is a space without boundaries, but found all over. Gold talks about loneliness in the city and the difference in feeling of belonging between countryside of childhood and city of now: *"No one belongs in London, and so everyone does. It is a community of not belonging"* (Gold, 2017, pg 5).

Loneliness is a symptom of an increasingly virtual and fractured world – so that even if we're together, we can feel alone. Dowling and Power (2012) explain that:

> . . . *temporal and spatial routines of individuals and families are increasingly fractured; family-centred home life is much more than family members spending time together doing the same activity, in the same space. The growing cultural valuation of individual needs and desires within family routines is manifest as a preference for individualised spaces within the home.*
>
> (Dowling and Power, 2012, pg 608)

In talking about boundaries of home-making and breaking real and imagined walls, Steiner and Veel (2017) talk of dividing walls: '. . . *home is often approached through a trite public/private dichotomy, emphasizing the walls of the dwelling as a dividing line'.* (pg 1)

These dividing walls don't necessarily need to be made of bricks and mortar. Indeed, Menary (2010) makes us consider the walls of our brains and asks us to reflect on where the mind stops and the rest of the world begins. This is an interesting psychological approach to ideas discussed earlier in this book, on social construction of place and identity, and later on authenticity and being our true self. A reasonably contentious debate in its own discipline, Menary (2010) considers whether the mind stops at the skin or whether it is externalised. We might then ask the question: could the mind be 'home' – does it extend beyond the walls of our brain? If the mind is extended beyond the brain walls, it could perhaps inhabit virtual worlds beyond the home walls too, be present there and here. The mind could be home and the home could be mind. In considering the implications of this for 'home screen' and presence at home even when the lights of the phone and computer are flickering – perhaps we can be present here and there, at home and in online worlds, extending the walls between mind and home.

The issue of loneliness isn't just a personal issue – there are societal impacts and costs, and there is a space for further exploration and intervention by state and charitable agencies. Harrison (2018) says, *"Loneliness is a social collective challenge that we need to face, but one that the NHS currently bears the brunt of".* Housing providers need to consider their role in combating loneliness. There are recent movements that recognise the growing problem of loneliness and sadness. Communities and charitable organisations are responding to the crisis of loneliness with a range of initiatives. Kindness.org is a social global movement which tries to respond to the unkindness that can be seen on the internet. Another movement, Camerados, started in Britain to help create friendships and a sense of purpose for people. Camerados offers some great initiatives such as 'living room in a box', as well as direct project work with the NHS where a space (a tipi) provides a place to recognise and share the feelings that can be amplified in situations like a hospital. The Jo Cox Foundation was set up to continue work on combating loneliness and isolation; work flowing out of that is shared with the global movement 'Common Ground'. If, as Harrison (2018) says, loneliness and isolation are collective challenges, then responses also need to be collective. Combating isolation, by its nature, cannot be a singular response – it needs to come from all of us. Part of that must be in recognising our shared humanity. No matter how many differences there may be in cultural and religious practices, between gender, age, fashion preferences, educational attainment, personality – there are more things that bind us. Quest for 'home' is one of those things that should bind us, but where the quest is individualised and overly marketised – housing rather than home focused – it can divide us.

Online worlds are an incredible global social connector. Bringing spaces to our home screen that we might otherwise never see. But connecting outside the home can reduce the connection within – we can end up alone, together. Turkle (2011) articulates this:

> These days being connected depends not on our distance from each other but from available communications technology. Most of the time, we carry that technology with us. In fact, being alone can start to seem like a precondition for being together because it is easier to communicate if you can focus, without interruption, on your screen. In this new regime, a train station (like an airport, a cafe, or a park) is no longer a communal space but a place of social collection: people come together but do not speak to each other. Each is tethered to a mobile device and to the people and places to which that device serves as a portal.
>
> (Turkle, 2011, pg 155)

What does this do to home? Home might be the world and the world might be home (as Gilman, 1903 wrote in her poem). However, it has the potential to weaken presence together in a physical place. Depending on our definition of self and place at any given time – our home screen can erode our home.

Conclusion

Social media and online space can be empowering virtual communities of support, protests for better governments and services – improved places. Online worlds can also be places to devalue domestic work, emotionally undermine and harm those physically isolated but connected online – but they can also offer virtual spaces of sisterly support and advice on domestic drudgery. Housing services online can provide more efficiency and consistency, but they can exacerbate loneliness for the tenant who used to have at least one human conversation a week with the rent collector. In the move to channel shift for efficiency, social housing organisations lose that capacity to be the 'always there' social support service. Traditional person-centred approaches to housing management allowed staff to notice symptoms of domestic violence, to see when a child may be at risk, to be a part of the solution to combating loneliness. Social and online communities can connect virtually, and appease isolation for those physically unable to get out and about. But they should be an addition to human connection, physical places – real-world experiences, not a replacement. Our homes – our walls – can physically screen us from the outside world, particularly as we saw in the previous chapter in gated communities. Our home screen on our computers and phones can also screen our identity by projecting an inauthentic performance of ourselves, our homes. Home already has a complicated intersection with place and identity – when we look at this through a lens of virtual online worlds, the notion of who we are and where we are present in place, becomes even more complex.

5 Precarious home

The challenge of homelessness

Introduction

According to UN Habitat data, 1.6 billion people worldwide have inadequate housing. Homelessness is a fast-growing symptom of poverty. For homeless people, this can lead to a series of devastating social, physical and mental health problems. This fifth chapter discusses the growing problem of homelessness. It is not just rooflessness, but includes the issues faced by Generation Rent and the problems of inaccessibility and unaffordability of a safe and secure home. Home is not just an individual entity where good governance stops at the front door. Housing as home, particularly, is so integral to our human rights that any caring society and its government should intervene when there is an absence of sufficient housing to call home.

Homelessness is on the rise across the UK. Figures show a year-on-year rise in street homelessness in recent times. The National Audit Office Report (2017) referenced national Department for Community and Local Government (DCLG) figures showing that: *"The number of rough sleepers stood at more than 4,000 in the autumn of 2016, having increased from fewer than 1,800 in the autumn of 2010"* (NAO, 2017, online). However, organisations like Shelter would argue this figure doesn't reflect the current reality. In a report published in November 2017, the organisation estimated 307,000 people were either sleeping rough or inadequately housed in Britain; the headline of their research was that this equated to one in every 200 people (*The Guardian*, 2017, online).

Who is homeless?

In some political and media discussions, 'the homeless' take on a presumed identity, they are othered and marginalised. Let's be very clear – homelessness is not a human characteristic, it is the symptom of policy failure and could happen to any one of us in certain conditions.

In her review of the literature, McNaughton outlined a typology of homeless dimensions:

1   *'Absolute' minimal homelessness – having no shelter at all, rough sleeping;*
2   *Homelessness pertaining to the nature or quality of the housing someone has;*
3   *Homelessness as it is subjectively experienced;*
4   *Homelessness as it relates to statutory definitions, or the welfare entitlement that exists surrounding housing in a given locale or time.*

McNaughton (2008, pg 4)

The European Federation of National Organisations Working with the Homeless (FEANTSA) and the European Observatory on Homeless developed a European classification of homelessness types (ETHOS). This typology also has shades of variation – although, it doesn't examine perspective (homelessness as it is subjectively experienced) like McNaughton (2008) does. The ETHOS types span across four conceptual categories: (1) Inadequate and (2) Insecure accommodation is classed as 'housing exclusion' and (3) houseless and (4) roofless, fall within 'homelessness'. There are critiques which question where exclusion stops and homelessness starts. Amore et al. (2011) suggest developments to the model based on classifications used in New Zealand and they moot four broad homeless categories: (1) without accommodation, (2) temporary accommodation, (3) sharing accommodation and (4) uninhabitable housing. These seem to reflect the lived reality of homelessness in its broadest sense. It is interesting to note the issue of sharing as a type of homelessness – when increasingly shared housing and co-housing models are part of projects proposing a solution (in light of affordable housing shortage, but also the benefits of sharing to combat loneliness, as we saw earlier in the book). Amore et al recommend that a further model of 'at risk' homelessness is created – not within the existing model but to sit alongside. Some of these risks can be seen in a typology of precarity, suggested momentarily in this chapter. Certainly with a growing private rented sector, lightly regulated and with relative insecurity of tenure, the group of people 'at risk' as well as the number of people already falling within the existing typologies, is getting larger.

It is important in understanding the full range of homelessness, that we understand the breadth of meaning of home. Homelessness as discussed by government and on the front pages of newspapers, then, is often 'rooflessness' – without the physical structure of a dwelling. But in the discussion on meaning of 'home' – the physicality of the dwelling – the house – is not the only ingredient in home; there is self-concept identity, connection with others (or not), isolation through the behaviour of others (controlling and violent behaviour of an intimate partner). This means that much homelessness is 'hidden' behind closed doors, in precarious and insecure housing – different entirely to rooflessness, but still requiring concern and intervention.

Housing precarity – homelessness risk

Beer et al.'s (2016) study on precariously housed people in Australia, found three measures of housing precarity: (1) housing costs in excess of 30% of income (this is a standard measure across housing studies of 'affordability'); (2) living in private rented accommodation (the authors explain that in Australia this tenure is insecure, which is in common with England but less so with other mainland European countries); and (3) the third measure in Beer et al.'s study was whether the survey respondent had been 'affected by a recent forced move'.

As with many of the concepts throughout this book, there is an aspect of relativity – to other people/ situations, and to alternative pathways or ideals in our own lives (how we perceive where are now to where we want to be). In an article (Richardson, 2017a) examining precarious housing as a way of explaining the liminality of Gypsy and Traveller accommodation, I suggested the following model:

- *Absolute precarity/adversity – based on measures of poverty or physical insecurity applicable to anyone, a static measure based on income, tenure type, physical environmental or health standards.*
- *Relative precarity/adversity – based on feelings of unfairness, where outcomes of poverty or physical insecurity are relative to others, such as comparative insecurity of tenure within one tenure type or one geographical area.*
- *Perceived precarity/adversity/fear – . . . An additional element of insecurity might be felt where all things considered there was a level of relative stability, but based on individual and in-group experiences both recent and historic, a level of anxiety and fear heightened notions of precarity, amplifying the effects.*

(Richardson, 2017a, pg 500)

This may be one aspect of considering Amore et al.'s (2011) recommendation to consider homelessness risk. It is important to remember that precarious and insecure housing, including relative precarity, is part of a spectrum of homelessness. Not without shelter to meet basic needs, but potentially on the edge of an accommodation precipice. The Homelessness Act 2017 recognised the need for intervention in this arena, sooner than the date on which a person is without a roof. The legislation required local authorities to prepare a plan, and to recognise earlier in the cycle of precarity, that this could lead to homelessness.

Millennial homelessness and the issue of ownership

Taking homelessness in its widest sense – beyond rooflessness – it is evident that there is a real impact of the difficulties in 'owning' a home, on younger people – Millennials/Generation Rent. The Resolution Foundation (2018) published the report of the *Intergenerational Commission* which told us that Millennials were facing higher housing costs and lower levels of home-ownership than their predecessors, and they also pointed to the issues of quality and security:

> *This rise in private renting means that young adults face greater housing insecurity than previous generations did. They are compromising on quality and convenience too.*
>
> (Resolution Foundation, 2018, pgs 11–12)

If the characteristics of a good and happy home – a feeling of being 'at home' – are related to affordability of cost, reasonable physical quality of the property, security of tenure; then younger people are being failed by a system that does not regulate for this sufficiently in a growing private rented sector which is increasingly the only channel through which young people are accessing accommodation. We are not providing them with ways in which to make 'home'.

Home-ownership is increasingly the preserve of those with wealth, or older people who bought at a time when housing was cheaper to buy. Some wealthier people own not just their own home, but they own an increasingly large amount of other people's homes – those renting in the private sector. The continued leverage of asset value and rental income creates the ability to purchase more homes to let, and so on. The private rented sector has grown at the expense of the social housing sector. Social housing has effectively eaten itself as the sector has been pushed towards so-called 'affordable' housing – which, at up to 80% market rents, just isn't affordable in many areas.

In other countries, in continental Europe – countries like Sweden – there is a different approach. The level of owner occupation is much lower; the private rented sector is better quality, more affordable and more secure for renters. But we are materially different in our political and economic systems and this manifests in the flavour of our housing markets. Kemeny (1995) highlighted the differences: in England, the private market is protected from competition through the suppression of 'cost' renting (social renting) – neo-liberal policies were the bedrock of this paradox in housing market approaches and this remains the case, more now than ever.

Pendulum politics, resulting from our democratic process, means short termism is the only political game in town. Reforming the housing market, fixing the private rented sector, building more genuinely affordable housing needs a longer term approach. Then there are voter dynamics to consider and elections to win; for example, Right to Buy (RTB) appeals to people already in the social housing sector who wish to own. It appeals as a political tool around elections, but it benefits the few, rather than the many, and it disproportionately disadvantages young people who are in the private rented sector and cannot benefit from RTB. Older people, those who own their own homes or wish to buy their council or housing association home, are more likely to engage with the current democratic system and vote. Until more and more young people use their ballot card, their voices will be marginalised, their housing increasingly precarious in a relatively unregulated private sector.

Homelessness across the globe

New York is renowned as the emblematic city in the land of opportunity. But, like many global cities, she has her share of housing crises. Street homelessness is still observable on many corners, but there have been some improvements in policy to reduce this. New York is unique in the U.S.A with a 'Right to Shelter' that aims to keep anyone who qualifies for accommodation under this scheme, off the street. But it is expensive, the rents and property values in New York, like London, mean that the unintended beneficiaries of such a policy are the private landlords who let properties for emergency shelter at premium prices. This diverts money from investing longer term into affordable bricks and mortar to house families now and for the future. There has also been a recent investigation which has shown the darker side of this – with poor, squalid conditions in some of the shelters. Whilst there may be fewer people physically sleeping on the street, the shelter 'industry' is sprawling.

Mayor Bill de Blasio focused on provision of more affordable housing as one of his key platforms during his first term. The New York City Mandatory Inclusionary Housing Policy (MIHP) Study (2015, pg 8) stated that *"The number of rent-burdened households in New York City has risen 11 percent since 2000, to almost 55 percent of all renter households"* (The policy defines 'rent-burdened' as families paying in excess of 30% of its income on rent – a truer reflection of affordability than the up to 80% of market rate definition in England). The MIHP was adopted at the end of March

2016, and it included relatively bold actions on numbers of affordable housing units to be included in new developments. However, there have been criticisms that it is not implemented fully, that developers are insufficiently monitored to see if targets are being adhered to. In England meanwhile, policies such as Section 106 planning gain agreements are also criticised – councils giving too much wriggle room to re-negotiate terms and targets for 'affordable housing' because of changes in 'viability' calculations.

On a work-trip to the U.S.A. in 2016, I revisited a project in New York which I had originally volunteered with as part of my senior year at high school in 1991. New York City Relief still offers individual support on the street in various locations across the city; volunteers take a bus equipped with hot soup and bread, water, clothes and first-aid. People offer some information on housing and employment, and there is also spiritual advice to help alleviate the 'hopelessness'. The charity was a little different from the one I volunteered with at school, but it still offered food and company for homeless people across the city. Charity like this can bring temporary relief and some spiritual hope to individuals that want that. But charity can't solve such a complex problem as homelessness, on its own, in the same traditional ways as it always has. Decades on, my more critically, reflective adult self could see the enormous good being done *to* and *for* homeless people on the streets of New York. But concerns nagged at the back of my mind about charities still there nearly 30 years on, still treating the same symptoms. Could it be more convenient, my less-charitable inner voice asked, for faith-based charities to save souls and reduce hopelessness in queues on street corners – than reaching into homes, opening doors? Did the visible presence of charity on the streets make government and society feel better about not structuring a sustainable solution to affordable housing and support shortage?

A flexible intervention at the systems level is required to solve homelessness. There is still space for charity and hope for homeless people on the streets, but structural government intervention, provision of affordable housing is required. Charity does not let government off the hook. In addition to the food, clothing, sleeping and hygiene apparatus, along with the faith and love so generously given by charities, there must be a wider more structured approach to help resolve the causes of homelessness – causes such as poverty and insufficient supply of housing. Affordable housing provision must be increased to meet need if we are to reduce and eventually stop homelessness, rather than just alleviate the symptoms of hopelessness. The no-nonsense answer to homelessness is the provision of housing with support.

New York city also gave us the 100,000 Homes Campaign, which won a UN World Habitat award in 2013. This 'Housing First' approach provides a sustainable home through a place to live, with support to recover from underlying issues. This is different to the traditional stair-casing model in England, where homeless people have been required to recover in hostels before they're seen as 'tenancy ready'. Flipping the model on its head is seeing success rates in homeless people getting into, and staying in, secure accommodation and there are a number of 'Housing First' models emerging across the globe, including a growing number in the UK.

World Habitat, the housing research charity which recognised the New York 100,000 Homes campaign with the UN Habitat award, have been following on with the campaign to end street homelessness, by sharing the principles from the project and supporting the *European End Street Homelessness* campaign. Leicester was one of the European cities which joined the campaign in 2017. In their 2016 return to DCLG, the city council in Leicester provided an estimate figure of 36 rough sleepers. There had not been an actual count or survey in the city for well over a decade. Charities led by Action Homeless, public agencies and De Montfort University (DMU) colleagues got together and decided the time was right to do something different. We decided to be in the vanguard of European cities who were taking part in World Habitat's European Campaign to end street homelessness. A key part of the campaign was 'Connections Week' in Leicester, which took place in November 2017. Ninety-three homeless people were surveyed in the city across the week. A prominent event during that period was the night-time street count, where over 80 students from De Montfort University got involved; thirty-one homeless people were counted on the night and several were able to take up the offer of hot food and a bed that night. The majority (95%) of homeless people interviewed had medium to high vulnerability scores. Homeless people in Leicester face multiple health needs with the most severe cases involving physical health, mental health and substance use issues. Forty per cent (40%) of respondents replied that their homelessness had followed a traumatic episode or experience.

Homelessness is a complex issue and requires a multi-layered partnership response. The campaign approach and methodology during 'Connections Week' seemed to work well and provided momentum for all the partners to continue working on the problem. Homeless people who answered the survey questions were provided with immediate sustenance and shelter that night, if they wanted to come in from the street – but longer term solutions are needed for those who have been through the 'revolving door' of hostels and street in previous homeless episodes.

Partnerships were of key importance to the Leicester campaign. Other cities have different innovations, and, say, in Manchester, they set out to use social impact bonds, to raise the funding necessary to house rough sleepers. Leicester partner agencies continue to meet and work together. One important aspect of the approach was to de-stigmatise homelessness, by bringing the people of Leicester into the campaign. This was something learnt from Community Solutions in New York in their 100,000 Homes Campaign. De-stigmatising people who are homeless, creates a stronger bond between residents and workers in the city and involves a range of different voices in the response – potentially reducing the occurrences of objecting to plans for new development.

Making 'home' without a house

So how do people make 'home' when they are homeless? There are strong emotional connections that are made amongst rough sleepers, there are ways in which people who are without even basic shelter, attempt to make themselves 'at home' where they are. Lenhard (2018) undertook research with homeless people sleeping in or around the Gare du Nord, asking about and observing their daily activities. Lenhard refers to this as 'core daily home making activity' through finding suitable shelter and preparing it – through the 'work' of making home. He refers back to Massey's (2005) concept of the constant changes in place – making and re-making itself, and he draws on this in explaining how the homeless people he saw in Paris, made and remade home, daily, in spaces in and around the train station. In the accounts of Lenhard's respondents, there are similar characteristics of 'home' on the street, as in house as home: relative security, cleanliness and ease of access. Walking through the city of Leicester, where I pass cardboard boxes laid out neatly, bags protecting pillow or other soft clothing, tucked under the top flap – I notice, the care with which items are placed, the daily ritual of trying to keep things safe, of staking a claim on the pavement or in the doorway. I think of this as I shake out my cushions on the sofa at my house – one of my daily rituals of making home tidy and welcome when I come back at the end of the day; and I think how lucky I am – and I know that we should all have shelter and a place to feel lucky at home.

Hostility: complicated responses to homelessness

Our public spaces are increasingly hostile. The conflict and negotiation of protecting home was explored, earlier in Chapter 3 of this book. Some of the complex issues around planning and negotiation can also help to frame our understanding of the messiness around responses to homelessness. On the one hand, there is a need to be good, to do good and help try to resolve homelessness. But on the other hand, there is often a negative or even hostile response to planning applications for more housing, particularly specialist homeless hostels. Many people seem to want to help homeless individuals, but not necessarily by saying yes to new homes – it's complicated.

Gentrification has not been a benign and harmless process; it has emptied city spaces of its poor and needy (Minton, 2009, 2017). Cities have also become less joyful and creative spaces to just be, to walk through, think and observe. The novelist Will Self joined a 'mass trespass' over recently privatised public spaces in the city, referring to how privatisation and closing off of space can affect us physically: ". . . it constrains imagination", he told Townsend (2016). City spaces have become much less accommodating spaces for homeless people to find a spot to sleep.

This built-in hostility is evident in the countryside in England too: bunded-up deep verges and lay-bys to stop Gypsies and Travellers from stopping (from travelling) in places they may have passed through for hundreds of years. Common lands that were once recognised as places that Gypsies would stay as they travelled for traditional work as the seasons changed, have been swallowed up as villages and towns have grown, or as traditional Vardos have been replaced by the white caravan and truck – less visually pleasing perhaps than the 'traditional ways' less palatable to settled communities. Of course, some encampments have and do cause trouble, leaving rubbish, bringing crime – but the response should be to those people for those incidents, rather than assuming it is a characteristic of a whole race of people and closing off places for them to live. In addition to the physical hostility of common spaces for Travellers, and more broadly for homeless people, there are policies and actions which have been brought in to 'protect' spaces from people. This can be seen, for example, in public spaces protection orders brought in by anti-social behaviour legislation in 2014. In some instances, these orders effectively create injunctions against a race of people, they disproportionately affect Gypsies and Travellers, for example.

Public spaces, open places in cities have been securitised through the use of hostile architecture. So-called homelessness spikes, poor doors, curved benches – all meant to keep the displaced and isolated apart from the 'us' in the city. Hostility to homeless people in the city is not the preserve of London and other global cities, it is evident across the world. Sahlin (2008) talked about the 'subtle' removal of benches, the closure of central blocks at night, and an anti-begging project in a number of cities in Sweden – all attempting to remove visible homelessness from the streets, particularly in gentrified areas.

Andreou (2015, pg 5) said:

> *Defensive architecture is revealing on a number of levels, because it is not the product of accident or thoughtlessness, but a thought process. It is a sort of unkindness that is considered, designed, approved, funded and made real with the explicit motive to exclude and harass.*

It may not be noticeable to people passing through a space at first glance, it is only when you need to sleep in a doorway or on a bench that you might notice the purposeful hostile design. It is purposefully designed though to protect the aesthetic of the city for those with vested interests (Petty, 2016). Those in power, with votes or through wealth, have an interest in clean streets, uncluttered by poor homeless people – so that they can attract investment. The global elite will not put their money into streets littered with sleeping bags and tents.

Nourishment and home

As noted earlier in this chapter, one way that a lot of people like to try and help is to volunteer with charitable projects which give out sleeping bags or hot food. Neither of these things is actively going to provide a house, which could be the basis of making a home, but they may make street homelessness temporarily more bearable. The giving of food, particularly, is a way of showing care, and doing good. Food and nourishment can make someone feel 'at home' for a moment. Many memories of home and family may relate to particular meals – flavours and smells. Nourishing, home-cooked food can go beyond filling the belly and reach our hearts too. Ezra – the fictional owner of the *Homesick Restaurant* in Tyler's (1992) novel – uses food to recognise and respond to emotions and feelings. If he thinks a customer needs the Okra soup, rather than the ham that was ordered, then that is what appears on the table.

The links between nourishing food and our feelings of being at home are complex. Nourishment may not happen in the family house – there are increasing levels of food poverty, a rise in the use of foodbanks and breakfast clubs. Across cities, a number of charities will provide food to help keep people from starving. One social enterprise in India – Akshaya Patra – has extended its help and support from the streets and schools of India, westwards to streets of England. Flipping traditional charitable geographies on its head, this Indian organisation is providing nourishing, carefully designed food, to poor students and to homeless people in London. The organisation recognises the need for nourishment – particularly for children in food poverty – who may have a roof over their head, but who are not getting the right kind of nutritional food to help them grow and flourish.

Food – good nutritional meals – is an important part of 'home' in the sense of being cared for, looked after and nurtured. Nourishing meals help a child to concentrate in school, achieve good grades and go on to meaningful and fulfilling employment. Where there is food poverty at home – where parents cannot afford to provide proper meals for their children – there is a need for social enterprise and charitable organisations to work together and to provide that support.

Conclusions

Housing and social policy is vital to a long-term strategic approach to homelessness in its broadest sense. We also need a rapid response and a 'housing first' type of approach to *ending street homeless*. Rather than leaving it to the market which has failed us and resulted in unacceptable rises in homelessness, we should aim for a government-led approach to halting the need for people to sleep on the street or sofa-surfing and other hidden homelessness. Homeless people have multiple and complex needs, as we found in our European End Street Homelessness project in Leicester. More and more people are sleeping on the streets. More and more young people are delaying their transition into adulthood by continuing to live in the parental home, or sharing with other people out of financial necessity when they may rather be moving in with a person they love, starting to build a family. An adapted 'housing first' type of approach (not a policy transplant, but a reflective look at how we can put housing at the focus of preventing homelessness) should be a next step. The appropriate response to homelessness – is to provide housing with some support for those that need it.

6 Home and away
Beyond bricks and mortar

Introduction

Housing, accommodation, takes form in all shapes and sizes. Some of it in solid granite, rooted in a place for centuries, some of it transient and temporary – a place where, also for centuries, a family has stopped to work and to meet others, for a time. In spite of the variety in physical form of 'home', there still seems to be an expectation that a home is made of bricks. In her protest folk song about 'little boxes', made particularly famous by Pete Seeger's cover version a year later, Reynolds (1962) highlighted an issue of conformity. If we didn't all go to university, play golf, get a management job and live in a 'little box', then we were not conforming to societal expectations. We need to consider alternative accommodation for 'others' (more broadly in society, but also physically in housing). This chapter will focus on 'others' and on appropriate accommodation for their cultural needs.

Home is more than the bricks and mortar of a house – it holds different meanings. For some, home is a base from which to perform and perhaps to travel from. Some of the arguments around provision of Gypsy-Traveller sites, and the misrepresentation of that culture relate to different imaginings of 'home'. When 'home' as a base has to be fought over though, the freedom to travel from and back to 'home' can seem like a distant dream. Additionally, 'home' to Gypsy-Travellers and other nomadic and Indigenous groups across the globe, may not be one place as a base, but instead a series of traditional spaces on a centuries-old route used by generations.

Housing conformity

I use the phrase 'housing conformity' in this book to highlight the ways in which our physical dwelling can suppress our identity, quash our creativity, wear us down and make us behave in a certain way – antithetical in some cases to a particular, traditional culture. Sometimes our accommodation, if it is seen to be different, imbues our identity and character in a certain way – it is a two-way process: us imprinting on the physical dwelling of home and home (re)shaping identity, sometimes in ways other than the way we wish to be seen.

In a lovely story which encapsulates how society creates conformity in how we view housing, from when we are young, Beadle (2007) tells us how he asked his four-year-old son to draw a house. After a long, tangential, creative line of questions, the boy clarified: *"Could it be the spookiest house in the whole of your world of men?"* (pg 3) and then proceeded to draw a fantastic multi-coloured creation with differing thickness of walls, and multiple chimneys. The next day – his first at primary school – Beadle's son came home excitedly at lunchtime having been asked to draw a house, with instruction from a teacher, it was:

> *a square box with four equidistant windows, rectangle in the middle, triangle on the top and a chimney from which smoke curled sky-wards. Len had entered the British education system, and the process of attrition through which the genius of children is mercilessly ground away had kicked in (with a vengeance) on the first day of his formal schooling.*
>
> (Beadle, 2007, pg 5)

The image of a house as square box made of bricks is learnt from an early age – it is the picture drawn by a million crayons, and it is the reality across hundreds of estates. Because the image is so strongly ingrained – anything that doesn't look like a variation on this box, is brought into sharp focus as 'other'. When this different-looking accommodation moves around because of nomadic habit, then that really is a threat of the 'other' (Richardson, 2006) to social sensibilities on housing and home.

'Non-traditional household types'

Oliver (2003) in his book, takes us across the world, and through his photographs and commentary demonstrates the breadth of different types of dwellings – going far beyond the square box made of bricks. Taking in nomadic and traditional lifestyles, he reminds us that home might be an igloo, a hut, a tent, a cave . . . different shapes and sizes, in towns, cities, deserts and seas. The different forms of dwelling are startling. There are very many nomadic cultures and people across the world. The Sami people travelling across Finland, Norway, Sweden and Russia today – herding Reindeer, crossing borders, following traditional ways, find themselves in conflict with settled people who find the grazing of the herds a nuisance.

Nomadic Fulani people in Africa herding cattle, also battling to access grazing land. The Roma, the Dom people, Inuits, Native Americans, Gypsies/Travellers and Aboriginal people – all with a nomadic heritage, trying to make and re-make home in places across the globe. And yet in the Western mind's eye, it is the box made of bricks which springs automatically to public consciousness.

In her work *Parklands*, Newton's (2014) research explores meaning of home with caravan dwellers (non-Travellers): people who live on mobile home parks. Newton's work takes place in Australia, but there are mobile home parks in abundance in the UK and in America and other countries. Mobile home parks can provide community and affordability – a sense of belonging. Certainly in the UK there are issues around security of lease and suitable regulation of park management which could create some level of insecurity. But caravan can be 'home', can fulfil those criteria which help to create a feeling of being 'at home'. Mobile home parks in the U.S.A. can imbue residents with negative stereotypes (insulting terms used in the U.S.A., for example, but which aren't so prevalent a negative discourse in the UK for non-Gypsy/Traveller residential caravan parks). The structure of the dwelling should not negatively define the inhabitants. Newton's work on caravan parks in Australia, and my own research on Traveller sites in the UK, should remind us that dwelling type is not necessarily identity. It may be an important factor where the accommodation type is crucial to keeping cultural heritage and traditional practices alive, but the type of property does not universally define the inhabitant. Not all Gypsies live in caravans, for example – not all caravans are 'home' for Gypsies.

Despres (1991) recommended that ". . . *the meaning and experience of home need to be investigated in the context of non-traditional household and housing types*" (pg 107). This part of the book aims to do just that, and it fills a gap in the current literature on 'home' by bringing in my understanding from research with 'non-traditional household types'; namely Gypsies and Travellers living on sites in the UK. It also draws on others', largely anthropological, work to reflect on nomadism and strong links to place (not bricks and mortar) in other 'non-traditional' households too.

Indeed, when we know we are dealing with 'other', we seem only to be able to do so in the extremes of caricature. 'Non-traditional households' seem to have to be so manifestly different, to mark them out as 'other'. For example, it is integral to the social, political and media imagination that 'real' Gypsies and Travellers, live in beautifully painted traditional, bow-top Vardos. In the wistful social construction of 'real' Gypsies, these old-fashioned caravans are drawn by horses, stopping in glades and dells in the countryside, the people undertaking traditional jobs and crafts. But caravans and modern vehicles are much easier to live in and travel with and so modern Gypsies and Travellers utilise vehicles and homes which have progressed with technology. This doesn't fulfil the public fantasy – we may recognise that the modern house has indoor toilets, electrical white goods to help us maintain 'home' – but we hold up stronger standards of tradition when it comes to 'others' like Gypsies.

This was also seen to be the case in Millard's (2018) documentary series, where it was revealed that members of the Korowai Tribe in West Papua had been asked to build tree-top housing for a previous documentary made in 2011. At the start of the (2018) programme, Millard explained that the Korowai people build tall houses in the trees because of physical dangers, but also because it was thought that 'Zombies and Witches' lived on the forest floor. Millard was told subsequently, when the homes were revealed as 'fake', that no one really lived in the tree-top houses; and moreover that the structure had been built to fulfil the imaginary of how it was thought tribe members lived, for the purposes of TV 'documentary'. He continued to try throughout the series to think critically about 'real' identity. Having thought that he'd found the last Korowai family to live in a tall house, without clothes, in a 'traditional way'; that even they were performing to meet the expectations of rich Westerners filming and at times, when they wanted to – they wore clothes. The 'trade' of identity was a key part of the modern Korowai economy, with families in town offering visitors an experience with various traditional activities. 'Traditional' or 'real' identities and ways of living, different-looking homes and dress are saleable commodities in the tourism economy and we are willing purchasers of this – even remotely through our televisions. The progress of modernity does not make such interesting viewing, even if it is 'real' and a reflection of the changes in places and identities, in response to technology and globalisation.

With both the Korowai and the Gypsy-Traveller examples – real modern day accommodation is different to the imaginary. It isn't a 'little box' but nor is it the traditional fantasmatic image (Richardson, 2006; Richardson and O'Neill, 2012). The result of this distance of fantasy and reality of image means that real people, in real (modern, affordable) mobile accommodation are not welcomed – plans are objected to, or people are moved out of traditional lands, because they fit neither the fantasy, nor the housing conformity.

Nomadism and home

There are many varied nomadic people across the planet; whilst their dwellings may each look very different, and whilst customs and daily practices vary – there are similarities of experience in connections between place, identity and home. This is something I have noticed in my research, talking to Gypsies and Travellers in the UK over the last two decades, and more recently in research with Indigenous people in Australia. Quicke and Green (2018) note similarities of experience across traditionally nomadic groups, within a 'politics of mobility': "*those peoples whose identities and lived experience are often contested through the interplay of population (im)mobilities and state regulation*" (Quicke and Green, 2018, online).

Aboriginal people in Australia are only recently telling their own story, their own identity, in their own way (Weedon, 2004). Historically seen through a white man's lens, the history of Indigenous communities in Australia shows an identity inseparable from the land and the sky, from the stories of ancestors. We can see similar experiences played out, for example, for Native Americans, whose ancestral links with the land and the earth have been undermined and undervalued in the fight against the oil pipeline in North Dakota. A number of tribes objected to the pipeline, including the Standing Rock Sioux Tribe living on the Indian Reservation in Dakota. The protest gave a global platform for some of the stories and voices about heritage, identity and connection with the land, but to no avail.

The Sioux and other tribes had a series of concerns about the oil pipeline in North Dakota, some of which aligned with wider environmental concerns around the potential for contaminating the river and water resources. The Trump Presidency signed an administrative order in 2017, and the pipeline was completed and became operational – overriding the protests of Standing Rock. Criticisms of the protest from industry and government figures aligned to the pipeline, were that other voices had joined the protest and that it had become an environmentalist, 'anti-oil' campaign – rather than strictly an objection from those on the land concerned about the impact of the pipeline on their home and their resources. Rather than the global concerns and connections with other people and groups joining to share in the fight, it was seen that the 'authenticity' of the objection had been hollowed out to become an empty signifier, to be used in the wider environmentalist protest discourse. In everyone being 'Standing Rock', the danger was that no one was seen as authentically fighting for the land. A similar situation occurred in the protest against the eviction of Travellers at Dale Farm – global attention was placed on the site, international film stars, UN human rights commissioners, all gave their voice. Anti-government, anti-austerity protesters joined the fight and physically chained themselves to the railings. However, in the widening base of protest to align with other movements – the authenticity of the protest again was undermined in the media and political discourse. Some physical sites of protest, like Dale Farm and like Standing Rock, become the focal point of global aims of protest – transcending the physical geographic location of their place. They become everywhere and nowhere. The globalisation of protest can impact negatively on the argument related to the physical place of home.

Barry and Porter (2011) examine the conflict inherent where traditional Indigenous groups, such as Aboriginal people in Australia, come up against a planning system rooted in White, Western legislation. They refer to the "contact zone" as an evocative method of framing the conflict-ridden debate on home and land rights. They go on in their later exploration (Porter and Barry, 2015) to show how discursive practices and processes can further marginalise and control Aboriginal people through limiting their rights and voices, further amplifying conflict in the contact zone.

Chatwin (1998) helps to frame an understanding of home and identity for Aboriginal people in Australia. 'Songlines' track the length and breadth of the country but are not visible to outsiders, they are known through song, landscape clues and link to the stars and memories of ancestors – stories passed down through generation after generation. Huge damage has been done through ignorance of culture, place and identity by settlers and modernisers who have built homes, diverted waterways, laid rail tracks and roads, devastating the song lines.

It is also interesting to reflect on the uneven impact of modernisation and cultural ignorance of Indigenous history, on different individuals in Aboriginal communities – for example the impact on men and women.

So what was it, I wondered, about these Australian women? Why were they so strong and satisfied, and so many of the men so drained?

(Chatwin, 1998, pg 102)

It is possible that in communities where the patriarchy has been particularly strong, that a modern world which devalues some of those traditionally male traits and trades will impact on a gendered basis. During research with Gypsies and Travellers in England, and then, following a visiting fellowship research project on housing disadvantage for Indigenous people, with my colleague Angela Spinney at Swinburne University to Australia – I reflected that in both communities the women seemed to have stronger voices, be more resilient, and more adaptive in leading change in modernity whilst still trying to preserve cultural heritage. This is an area I continue to research – rich for more detailed exploration. The housing disadvantage research in Australia included a series of focus group interviews with Aboriginal tenants and with professionals working in specialist Aboriginal housing advice and advocacy organisations. The stories from the tenants, the loss felt – not just in their own lives, but for generations past: impacting on generations future – brought us to tears. As researchers, we sympathised with the trauma of the disadvantage felt, every day – the poverty and isolation, the sense of loss of identity and connection. We also observed the careful work being undertaken by the advice and advocacy organisations working with people who had complex and entrenched needs. There are a number of similarities noted in Aboriginal community and Gypsy/Traveller people. For example, cultural practices around children of the opposite sex after a certain age sharing living and sleeping quarters in proximity. Some traditions around grieving have similar (not same) implications around the need for flexibility around the home and housing management. Both communities need links with outdoors, land, sky, family connections – this too has implications for creating and managing home, especially in modern urban environments.

Intersections of different identities in different places create issues of conflict that can result in violence and internally displaced people. There are a number of examples of this across the globe, ranging in severity and complexity. This history of internal displacement of people is horrific and murderous, it still happens today. The Ogu at Otodo-Gbame community in Lagos are one modern-day example, where the authorities were allegedly witnessed setting fire to the homes along the water's edge and driving people into the water (Osman and Busari, 2017). It is seen with the suspected genocide of Muslim Rohingyas in Myanmar (Nebehay and Lewis, 2018). This is happening now – still. It is also seen closer to home, in recent years in Europe, with the forced eviction and removal of Roma camps in a number of countries (Richardson and Ryder, 2012). Even closer, the internal displacement of people, in most cases less violent, it is happening in England, with the eviction and constant movement of Gypsies and Travellers from 'unauthorised encampments'.

Indeed, whilst this part of the book is looking at nomadism and home, it can be seen that poor people – nomadic or not – are being displaced from cities. Sometimes this is movement from council tower blocks that are being refurbished as part of renovating the city; but which results in displacing residents for years and disrupting the community beyond repair. It is rare for a housing association to deliver the social housing aspects of a renovated area first, because of the economic and viability appraisal – profits from the market sales are said to be needed for delivering the 'affordable' housing. But some housing associations are looking to turn this model on its head so that poorer people, those who cannot afford market rent or sale, are not completely displaced from their community, from their social identity.

Gypsies, Travellers and Roma

There are examples in Europe where Gypsies, Travellers and Roma face extremely high levels of discrimination. I visited Bucharest in 2015, on the invitation of the British Embassy in Romania, to take part in a human rights debate focusing on representation of Roma in the media. As part of my trip, I visited Bucharest Sector 5 – the Ferentari 'ghetto' (an extreme example of the impact of discrimination) to see for myself the living conditions of Roma in the area, and to speak to some of the inspiring people working with families to improve educational outcomes. Extreme poverty was manifest in the area: lack of water and electricity in many properties, evidence of drug use amidst piles of rubbish. An angry-looking man with an axe in a shopping trolley approached me and my companions – a nerve-wracking moment on the face of it – but it transpired he had no heating in his flat; he was going to chop wood to burn to keep warm, first appearances being deceptive in this scenario. Amidst the poverty and the cold, I met children, teachers and parents full of hope, clearly 'at home' in an area which at first glance was a desperate place. The residents and teachers in Sector 5 that I met were frustrated at the discrimination and negative perception of Roma in Romania; and indeed, in conversations with non-Romanian Roma I heard some extremely derogatory comments. Words are never just words: they translate into policy and action which can discriminate (Richardson, 2006) and which was writ large in the housing conditions I saw.

Gypsies, Travellers and Roma are subject to discrimination in the UK too, particularly in the way they are spoken about in public, media and political debates.

One neat way of examining the severity of this problem in public discourse is to apply a method that journalist Jake Bowers has used to highlight this issue. Replace the word Gypsy, Traveller or Roma with any other recognised ethnic group, and see if it makes you wince. Here is just one example to try this method – a Westminster Hall debate on 10 June 2015: "Effect of Gypsies and Travellers on local communities". The very title of the debate alienates whole ethnic groups, seen – not as part of local communities, but instead affecting them. Some aspects of the actual debate underlined extremely negative perceptions of Gypsies and Travellers, but there were also MPs who sought to bring balance and to highlight the negativity of the prevailing discourse.

What politicians say, and how they say it, has an impact on how they implement ideas and policies. In Moore and Coates v Secretary of State for Communities and Local Government (2015) the secretary of state was found in breach of the Equality Act 2010 as a result of indirect discrimination due to the 'call in' policy applied to all planning appeals related to Gypsy and Traveller sites in the green belt. The Secretary of State was found to have breached article 6 of the European Convention on Human Rights. And it isn't just in political actions where discriminatory practice can be found. In the case of the Traveller Movement and others v JD Wetherspoon (2015), the pub chain was found to have racially discriminated against Gypsies and Travellers after staff refused them entry to a pub in London. These actions by government ministers, by the entertainment industry and by the media are not surprising – they are physical manifestations of a much wider negative discourse.

The negative discourse creates a hostile social context, which creates reactionary moments (bans, evictions), which creates further negative discourse – and so on. Public political discourse makes its way from the Cabinet in Whitehall, to the social conversations around our kitchen tables. The negative discourse creates a climate of fear and a culture of 'no', of blocking off common spaces for temporary stopping. Noor (2018) questions how she can challenge the vehement objection to Travellers stopping on common land, having noted a recent securitisation of a common in her area where Travellers have traditionally stopped in the past. We need more political leadership, from cabinet ministers to local parish councillors, to improve the tone of public discourse on Gypsy and Traveller issues, which affects planning for sites, but also their treatment more widely in society.

The voices of Gypsies and Travellers themselves need to be heard more too, so we can all talk about a shared understanding of the meaning of home – whatever home looks like for each of us. In a small project with Rooftop Housing and other progressive housing providers, during 2017 and 2018, I worked with poet Damien Le Bas and a young film-maker, Polly Garnett, along with members of Gypsy and Traveller communities who shared their voices and their photographs to tell about the meaning of 'home' for them. It transpired that if you listen, there is so much more that is common to us all in 'home' – security, a place to be yourself, to connect with family and loved ones, to access services such as doctors, schools, social spaces.

Definitions make a material difference

How people are defined by the state and how they define themselves will differ. In some cases the definition by the state can have a severe impact on employment, housing, poverty. The Windrush scandal in 2018 showed that without the paperwork – the official government recognition of definition as British citizen – people were being denied healthcare, they were let go from their jobs, they had difficulty accessing housing; some faced physical deportation. Although here for decades: part of their community, state definition for the Windrush generation in Britain was crucial. We can see this in the history of Australia for Indigenous Aboriginal people – without official recognition even of their humanity, they were not seen as people of that place – centuries of living a nomadic life on the land, ignored. It is also possible to see the impact of definition today in the U.K.: particularly complex around nomadism. New planning definitions which came into force in 2017 requiring those who considered themselves as ethnic Gypsies and Travellers to demonstrate – for planning purposes – that they lived a nomadic life for economic reasons. Ongoing research shows that the impact of the emerging implementation of this definition, through analysis of Gypsy and Traveller Accommodation Assessments, appears to show a relatively low proportion meeting the new planning definition. This has implications not just for self-identity, but will have practical impacts on the delivery of sufficient sites for all Travellers to live on.

The antagonistic forces within a discourse are fluid and not fixed; differences can be constructed and reconstructed. If we think about the social construction of Gypsies and Travellers in the social space, we can see the construction of identity which creates antagonistic communities, and yet the identity is not fixed but constantly changing. Think of the example of public, press and politicians blaming Gypsies and Travellers for their own lack of accommodation and place in the community because of an 'unwilling-ness' to settle and live as the rest of society, in houses. However, when talking about Gypsies and Travellers who have bought a plot of land and applied for planning permission to allow them to live that settled life demanded by public, press and politicians, in order to be accepted as part of society; they are then seen as not 'real' Gypsies and subsequently threatened with having their racial and cultural identities stripped away (this removal of cultural identity upon settling is enshrined in planning law, but not so in equalities legislation). If Gypsies and Travellers, having been made homeless through being moved on from roadside encampments persistently, move into a house as the only option offered by a council in response to a homeless application, they are seen as not needing a site or roadside accommodation (even if they are included in an accommodation needs assessment, their desire to be on a site rather than in a house may be seen as *preference* rather than *need*). Fewer sites are built, more Gypsies and Travellers have to go on the roadside, they are moved on and on, and on, perhaps they eventually move into housing – but they are still seen as 'other' even when they conform, or are coerced to conform. This seems to embody the articulation (and re-articulation) within antagonistic discourse practices. There is always conflict involved, sometimes overt, but sometimes implied, but there is no fixed boundary to the antagonistic practices, or the groups party to this process of power and control. In other words, if rules and group identities are fixed then it is possible to learn the rules and engage in resisting the dominant power; but if the rules and identities are constantly changing and being re-articulated then resistance is much more difficult.

In his (1991) work, Bordieu discusses identity, representation and meaning; which is helpful in understanding perceptions of marginalised groups:

> *What is at stake here is the power of imposing a vision of the social world through principles of di-vision which, when they are imposed on*

a whole group, establish meaning and a consensus about meaning, and in particular about the identity and the unity of the group, which creates the reality of the unity and the identity of the group.

(Bordieu, 1991, pg 221)

This can be seen in the 'di-vision' that occurs in the spatial segregation of the location of 'non-traditional' housing, such as Gypsy/Traveller sites, and in some cases their neglectful management (Richardson and Codona, 2016). The power of the dominant majority community, through the imposition of supposed identity, is evident in words, but also is physically evident in poor management of some council sites. Whilst it is important that groups should self-define rather than have external labels imposed, there is a challenge over 'ownership' of a label and also fixity with a wider discourse.

As Atkinson and Jacobs (2016) say: *"Space and place are important because the households we comprise are affected by qualities and amenities of specific locations"* (pg 110). Habitus in this regard may be similar to Foucault's (1967) 'heterotopia' – a segregated set of ideals that protect the community from the norms of wider society which are seen as a threat to traditional Traveller ways. The segregation is often place-based, there are barriers and boundaries to sites to stop non-Travellers encroaching, and to an extent, the segregation is self-selected. But it is not as simple as that. From analysis of over 400 planning appeal decisions (Richardson, 2011), the majority where permission was granted included conditions related to 'screening' of the new site – literally a requirement for the site to be *hidden* behind landscaping. The segregation in place is something that settled and Traveller communities promote; the latter, though, need the boundaries to be highly permeable so as to integrate into schools and to conduct trade but it is this which can be problematic, particularly where the physical place is on the outskirts rather than within community boundaries.

Piazza (2014) finds in her study of Irish Traveller women in Brighton that 'place' is more than physical. For example, she suggests that the women can feel loyalty to 'home' the place in Ireland where they were from, as well as to the place they were currently residing in, and that the loyalty to the current space was not just about physical attributes:

for these travellers, place means something more than a physical location. Instead of a geographical reference point, the women's locality is identifiable with the affordances that make these disenfranchised travellers' lives liveable – for instance, electricity, taxi rides to school or the play bus with children's books.

(pg 271)

However, clearly, in that moment of location the physical space, the ability to protect family on a well ordered site away from the threats of the rest of the world is of huge importance. The notion of a 'placeless' Gypsy is a persistent myth (Kabachnik, 2010b) and perhaps because of this perception of them being without place there is a wider public imagining that they therefore 'invade' 'our' places (Kabachnik, 2010a).

Liminal spaces are physical and psychological places where identity is constructed and recreated by individuals themselves, by wider communities and by the state. The impact of the re-creation of these liminal spaces – in the physical and social imagination forms – is one of insufficient accommodation for Gypsies and Travellers – physical and social accommodation in the widest sense. Our public discourse – from the kitchen table, to the Commons benches and in our newspapers and online articles – creates a debate which sees no place for temporary use of public spaces to accommodate Gypsies and Travellers (in a way that has been acceptable in previous centuries when nomadic trades-people were seen as essential to support local economies or to entertain people). More and more places are bunded-off to prevent homeless people sleeping on park benches (McVeigh, 2016) or Travellers stopping for a while on a deep verge or corner of a common land.

Sharing common land

Common land, is sometimes seen as belonging to everyone, but sometimes to no one. It can be the source of conflict when put to an alternative use, or where one person's use prevents another's. As has been discussed earlier in this book, common land in cities and in the countryside is increasingly formalised or securitised. There are relatively few informal spaces that can be used 'meanwhile'. One example of 'meanwhile' use was given in the introductory chapter, a managed risk approach to the building site of St Clements Hospital as part of the East London Community Land Trust development – when space was used for a community cafe, a summer festival, play areas, community project spaces. The London Plan in 2017 has formalised the idea of 'meanwhile use' – including statements of land supply for potential temporary stopping places and sites. Plans need implementing, however, and informal approaches are difficult to regulate.

There have been attempts over centuries to share land, so that resources don't wither from overuse, and so that there is equity in use across different claims. There are a range of models that can be examined for common land sharing (Buck, 1998), and indeed decision-making and power sharing. Ostrom (1990) pays attention to methods, such as the Turkish fishing sites rota which draws on collective action to share Common Pool Resources

(CPR) and she provides some design principles for sustainable regimes on sharing the commons:

- Clearly defined boundaries
- Operational rules congruent with local conditions
- Collective choice arrangements
- Monitoring
- Graduated sanctions
- Conflict resolution mechanisms
- Minimal rights by government to challenge sustainable regimes
- Nested enterprises (particularly for larger systems).

Ostrom didn't argue that the principles were all necessary, or sufficient, to support CPRs. As part of Gypsy and Traveller accommodation assessment and other evaluation research, questions around community land trust approaches for permanent site provision, housing co-operative frameworks have been mooted as alternative approaches, but not yet resulted in particular schemes. There are ideas that have been successful around meanwhile use of common land for temporary stopping places negotiated with local authorities. A number of informal arrangements are in place, along with more publicised approaches, such as the Negotiated Stopping approach in Leeds.

Conclusion

We must go beyond house as home in order to get a better understanding of the meaning of home and the intersection of place and identity. Moreover, we should also move past the ingrained notion of house as dwelling. There are many different dwelling types from tent to trailer, from igloo to tree-house. By restricting the public imaginary to a box made of bricks, we exclude all other dwelling types as 'other' – as a threat. Indeed, we then socially construct identity characteristics according to a fantasy of what sort of people must live in a place that doesn't look like our own. This creates a framework of housing conformity, which excludes and denies varied cultural traditions and practices, marginalising identities, banishing them from places and spaces. Through a recognition of the negative impact of political, social and media discourse on marginalised groups – on people with traditional nomadic ways of life, we can hold politicians and newspapers to account – challenge the hegemonic exclusionary debate. We can examine different ways of sharing common land by recognising the conditions that could be in place to make the arrangement sustainable and fair.

7 Home is in the heart

Authentic self and identity

Introduction

Home is a place where the journey to authenticity can happen, when that home is allowed, and supported, to be a nurturing space. This book has tried to explore some of the reasons why 'real' is difficult – real me, real home. If real home is a place to perform our authentic identity, there are many challenges along the way. Some of the challenges explored so far in the book are around construction of meaning, of ourselves, of neighbours, of home. This can be diverted or thwarted by the reconstruction of others, by social, media and political discourse defining and redefining people and places. It can be derailed through legislation which recognises people as real, only if they define in a way that fits our imaginary – Travellers who are traditionally nomadic, for example.

Really authentic?

Our identity and authentic self is wrapped up in home – either our current dwelling if that 'feels like home' or some other place or time. This chapter questions how home might be in us, rather than us in home. Trinkets relating to 'home' or culture, held with us, can help to remember who we are to reinforce our authentic identity and, where we don't live 'at home' in our current dwelling place, can make life more bearable. It also debates how the 'heart' and the 'head' can be in conflict in social housing organisations who, in response to austerity, find their central mission in question.

Agreeing on a definition of 'authenticity' is challenging. Definitions are not just the written or spoken word, but the lived experience, the social construction of people and places in practice. Lindholm (2008) attempts to explore the meaning of authenticity:

> there are two overlapping modes for characterizing any entity as authentic: genealogical or historical (origin) and identity or correspondence

(content). Authentic objects, persons, and collectives are original, real, and pure; they are what they purport to be, their roots are known and verified, their essence and appearance are one . . . these two forms of authenticity are not always compatible nor are both invoked equally in every context, but both stand in contrast to whatever is fake, unreal, or false, and both are in great demand.

(pg 2)

In his examination of the origins of our attempts at understanding authenticity, Lindholm (2008) debates the contribution of Rousseau in the eighteenth century, which took a confessional approach to revealing ones' essential self as a true good. His *Social Contract* (Rousseau, 1762) attempted to bring together the individual need to 'be' one's authentic self, within wider societal rules and laws. But this is the rub – we are only our self in relation to the place we're in. We need to be ourselves, but within a space. If authentic self is the pathological need to be truthful – come what may, to reveal our innermost self at all times, then creating home – negotiating home – allowing others to have their home, would be impossible. Within the home there is duty which isn't truth – domestic and other chores which if truth left untrammelled would not be done. If performing authenticity is achieved through revealing all ultimate truths and living them to the full, then negotiation around sharing space, creating places would not occur. So, there needs to be an exploration of self and home, which goes beyond the walls of the mind and the walls of the house – home is then a village, a town, a city, a country, a continent, a planet. Self is a community of people perhaps looking for a place – together or perhaps separate but accepted in that place. At the core of this – who are we, me? Where are the boundaries of home, place?

But we know the definitions are ever changing – contextualised by time and space, within the bounds of others' expectations of themselves and us. The meaning of home – our home – to us – changes depending on a great number of factors. So if we're challenged to define our own self, or own home, there is no wonder that taking the abstract to the particular and concrete, looking at actual policy to try to 'deliver homes' for those that need housing, is a challenge indeed.

The difficulty in defining and redefining self is also found in the expectation of a 'performance' of authenticity which fits an ideal. 'Performance' as an art form, as theatre (rather than performance as undertaking a function – performance of an athlete, a car) was examined in the early part of this book. In my research on accommodation for Gypsies and Travellers over the last two decades, it has been apparent that Travellers are expected to 'perform' a version of authenticity which has been socially constructed on the basis of nostalgia and fairytale. 'Real' Gypsies live by the campfire in a bow-topped wagon, I've been told by others who will have interacted with many 'real'

Gypsies but not necessarily known about it. We know that Gypsies and Travellers have modernised, with modern caravans, or living in housing – they don't look like the fairytale, but they are still 'real'. To meet expectations, to get to where they need to be – there may well be performance. There may be 'passing' (Silverman, 1982), either through hiding identity to get employment or indeed amplifying aspects of identity – dress, caravan and crystal ball, for example – to earn money through fortune telling for example – through a performance through show, which meets others expectations of 'authenticity'.

As seen in chapter three, the very act of being observed (or being thought to be observed) affects behaviour (Foucault, 1977). This was shown explicitly in Millard's (2018) television documentary on the Korowai. In the first of three episodes, the 'real' Korowai people were shown first to retain their hunter-gatherer roots – living in houses in the trees, unclothed, catching prey with spears, speaking Korowai rather than Indonesian – retaining their historic culture. Millard specifically wanted to see the 'real' Korowai people, and he revisited several times, to see how they lived throughout the year. Through this method, he was able to see that on return for the second visit, there had been a performance. The majority of Korowai people had moved to towns with government built basic wooden houses (and it was suggested this may have been to clear the forest of people to sell land and logging rights). Nakedness was a thing of the past apart from the two older men, who still lived in their tree-house until it fell down in the final episode. Younger Korowai people wore modern clothes when they could obtain cash to buy them – the ubiquitous football shirt loved by kids across the globe. The performance in fact was shown to be explicit and an essential part of the tourist industry. Korowai knew to take their clothes off and go to the forest to perform for foreigners – to live the traditional way. But when the foreigners went home, so did the Korowai.

What Millard showed was not just the performance of traditional ways for foreigners, but the emerging internal struggle for authentic self. If the hunter-gatherer ways were over, what role was there for the Korowai – what should they do, how should they be? The documentary tried over the last two episodes to show this, but what was reflected back was the ongoing struggle of the people themselves to know who they were, where home was, what and who they should be. The act of observing through the television cameras, had, as Millard accepted, altered the very performance (as function rather than theatre) of home and self. Whilst the programme showed us very extreme edges of this sphere of exploring self and home, it has the effect of amplifying our own struggles with the very same questions – who are we, and what is home?

Belonging and balance (at home at work)

Gilman (1903) suggests that home is where the heart is – where we can find peace. But this is a truce perhaps, a negotiated way of being for now. A balance between the love and duty of home: an agreed pathway between historic traditional ways, and finding our place in the modern world. Brown (2010) asks us to think about 'belonging' as part of identity and self. Indeed, 'home' is that sense of belonging, either in a physical place – house as home – or by being with a community of people who understand (as can be seen in some of the complex responses to entrenched homelessness, earlier in the book in chapter five).

> *Belonging is the innate human desire to be part of something larger than us. Because this yearning is so primal, we often try to acquire it by fitting in and by seeking approval, which are not only hollow substitutes for belonging, but often barriers to it. Because true belonging only happens when we present our authentic, imperfect selves to the world, our sense of belonging can never be greater than our level of self-acceptance.*
>
> (Brown, 2010, pg 26)

Let us take into consideration that 'home' can be in multiple locales – belonging and home could be with a school community, a street homeless community, it is not necessarily restricted by geographical space. Home might also be at work – the ability to be one's authentic self, to be happy undertaking tasks related to employment, requires a value alignment between individual and employer. If one is to feel 'at home, at work' then authentic values and aims need to work together. The social housing sector – the profession which aims to help support the finding of 'home' for those excluded from the housing market – has itself been going through an internal battle over values – a fight between the head and heart in profession. But of course, in reality, this has been much more nuanced than traditional binary debates in the public sector on 'commercial – bad/ social – good'. In research undertaken for the Chartered Institute of Housing (CIH) (Richardson et al., 2014), people were keen to find ways of expressing 'commercial' as 'business for a purpose' and certainly tenants who spoke to us saw themselves as customers and wanted better accountability as 'customers'. Le Grand (2013) responds to the squeamishness in the use of markets/ commerciality through the discussion of anthropological experiments showing that participants are more disposed to sharing resources in a market based system compared with non-market societies. He attempts to show the need for a market system to allow people working in public services to act as knights (working for the public good) rather than knaves. In other words, the presence of a market (of commerciality per se) does not drive us all to be knaves motivated only by self-interest. So, in terms of social housing – the notion of a commercial approach need not be at the expense of maintaining our social heart, but indeed our social heart may be better maintained with a commercial head. But it is difficult to see this in the realm of austerity and the impact of welfare reform on tenants.

The CIH research (Richardson et al., 2014) found that 'commercially minded' housing organisations needed to recognise and find balance with social values. An organisation which achieved that balance: 'Business for a purpose', not selfish profit, but creation of surplus for reinvestment in genuinely affordable housing and support, might look like:

- an organisation-wide dedication to maintaining financial sustainability
- relational rather than transactional ways of working with tenant-customers
- co-production methods: prepared to work with and alongside customers
- an understood context of firm, fair and managed boundaries
- a strong commitment to achieving outcomes
- a willingness to automate, adapt or discard processes, but retain human connection where it matters
- intelligence-led in terms of priorities and effort – investing time where it is needed
- pre-emptive action and proactive problem-solving (the traditional balance between planned maintenance and responsive repairs, but applied across all functions of housing and support, as a business ethos)
- a focus on long-term sustainability of the organisation, of the tenancies, of community
- empathy with customers – reflected in practices
- commitment to helping customers to address and resolve the difficulties they sometimes face – for example through 'coaching' approaches to housing patch management
- a flexible but proactive and firm approach to problem-solving – not leaving difficult issues, but getting involved in order to help, acting on observations of potential domestic violence, for example.
- investment in customers to gain life skills and develop self-sufficiency – working with, not doing 'to' or 'for'
- constructive working with local partners – linking with health, education and other services
- capturing efficiencies that don't negatively impact on customers wherever possible – genuinely better ways of working, not neo-liberal cuts hiding behind a community co-production face

(Adapted from Richardson et al., 2014, pg 36)

But finding the social housing sector's self, its values, is not simple. The social housing sector currently seems to be fighting to find its identity and retain a balance between heart and head. Wrapped up in this industry self-reflection, is the tenant (customer) who is bearing the brunt of increasing austerity and state-retreat at a time when the market is not offering sufficient affordable and secure housing. Frontline housing work is changing and diversifying within an industry that isn't precisely sure about 'who' it is.

In ongoing research to follow up the CIH Frontline Futures project, I've been examining vicarious pain and resilience of those in the sector – those feeling the pressure of these changes and the identity dilemmas that frame them:

> *Front line housing roles have always been pressured but now it is heading down an unprecedented path. With welfare reform, budget changes and government requirements of housing associations things have changed. The nice to have services, like subsidised decorating for elderly customers is disappearing. Tenancy support is extremely difficult to source now. Whilst we are pushed to be more commercial we aren't on a level playing field with the private sector. Our customers often have complex needs and aren't able to self-serve or carry out tasks independently. Our involvement with other agencies is also more pressured as we all try and protect our decreasing budgets with less staff than we previously had.*
>
> (Respondent 12, anonymised, 2016a)

The pressure of the challenge facing the tenant-customer can be harrowing, but it is the constraint in not being able to find a solution, refer to a further support service, which can cause internal dilemma and vicarious pain for the housing worker. The heart of the social housing sector is, still, a vital part of its self-identity, the head (driven by budget cuts) pulling away – creating tension. Organisations are looking back at the original values of their founders. For example, Peabody Housing, in early May 2018, announced that it would freeze or cut rents for around 4,000 of its properties. The argument in the public sector about what is 'affordable' in terms of housing costs, has been ongoing since the term was changed in housing legislation, meaning provision was turning from social housing (closer to 50% of market value) to so-called 'affordable' housing (closer to 80% of market value – making rents distinctly unaffordable for many). The critical reflection on the impact of the turn from 'social rent' to so-called 'affordable' rent is refreshingly welcome and more reminiscent of the original intent and values of the founder of the organisation – George Peabody. It would be welcome to see this as the start of a sector-wide move, led by the large organisations with strong charitable, social value, heritage.

In the creating, consuming and providing of home, the balance between self and community, between head and heart, is a vital part of understanding and reflecting our identity – of being 'at home' in where we are and what we do.

Home is in the pocket (or drawer or shelf)

Open our office drawers and it is possible that lurking in there are small trinkets, photos, a misshapen piece of child-made pottery, that help remind us of home, and, therefore, of who we are. Important trinkets that can help in times of uncertainty and pressure at work: that vital piece of home in the heart – linked to 'home' rather than current location. During a challenging day at work, it might soothe to look at a photo, pick up a mug from home or some other trinket and to feel the calm of home, at work, in that moment. Physical objects make our home – they don't just decorate home, they reflect moments and memories of family, or past adventures. This element of home in the objects that we collect can make important considerations around 'down-sizing' difficult. Incentivising/penalising tenants who live in a house too big for them, but for which either the physicality of the place is the memory or the objects stored within – such objects are not 'mere things', they are home.

The complexity of feelings about home, and being at home, can be invoked by home-related objects. The love and duty of home, in the objects we keep, can provoke strong feelings of guilt as well as feelings of love. When my son was very small and in thrall to the adventures of Harry Potter (Rowling, 1998), he saw me at the table on my laptop working late (again) and – half annoyed/half sad – he handed me his little sock and explained that, as Harry Potter does for the enslaved house elf Dobby, my son was freeing me from work. To this day, I keep the sock – in a place out of view, but readily within reach. Sometimes I forget it is there and when I accidentally touch it, in the pocket of my bag, I flashback to the wet-eyed, thick-throated feeling of guilt and love I experienced in that original moment: of not being present at home, being distracted by work. I still do it – work from home when I really shouldn't, come home from the office some days later than I should – it is a relief from the duty of home; and home is a relief from the job. My work is part of me, an important aspect of my identity: I find my job (mostly) interesting and engaging. But I adore my home and the people in it – it is a place of love and support and I know I take it for granted. All this feeling in a tiny sock – feelings of home: love and duty.

Connected self

Thinking about 'oneself', understanding what we mean by authentic self – identity and belonging in a place – home, is a challenge. As we've seen, the construction of identity of individuals, communities, people and places, is subjective, and it is contextualised temporally and geographically. The words and images we use to describe ourselves and others are part of the discourse of identity and place – the social construction of 'home'. Some of the words and definitions used are on a spectrum, seen as ranging from 'good' to 'bad'. Self is one such word. If someone called me 'selfish' I would not feel good about how I was perceived – to be seen as looking after myself above others: selfish is 'bad'. If I was called selfless, that could be seen to be necessarily 'good' – altruistic and caring: putting others' needs above my own. Selfishness though – looking after oneself, means others don't need to, saving money from communal budgets, preventing others worrying, because I'd looked after myself – couldn't that be good? But 'self-ish' can also lead to prohibitive individual gains (wealth held by the richest 1%), gated communities, isolation, disconnection and loneliness. Selfless-ness, if we were being literal and using a depressurised airplane as context, could lead to a delusional hypoxic state and death for anyone who hadn't 'selfishly' put on their own oxygen mask first – we'd try to be everywhere but ending up nowhere.

Finding the balance between 'ish' and 'less', in relation to self, is challenging. There isn't a satisfactory word or phrase which fits the gap. 'Self-connectedness' is possibly the closest description, for a comfortable point in this balance. The self isn't less or more, but is constantly maintaining whilst finding its connection with place and with others. It focuses on the feeling of being authentic self in connection with place and others, not on the process of connectedness. Where is this balancing and re-balancing between 'ish' and 'less' likely to occur? At home – whether a physical structure, or a social group – home is where we find and balance self and its connections. Home is our root of self which connects then with other roots in wider community and society. Nepo (2018) reminds that we may seem different on the surface but that together we are better, more resilient and connected at the roots, than we are alone.

Conclusion

The quest for home is a search for belonging and balance at the intersection of place and authentic identity. Understanding what we mean by 'authentic' within a framework of performance of home is challenging. And yet it continues to be important to examine the characteristics and conditions to create home – for us all. This could mean understanding how to look at common land and create a framework for sharing. It certainly means understanding how home manifests elsewhere – in objects, or in the matching of individual values and organisational goals in our workplace. Understanding who we are is not necessarily selfish, it is worth continued exploration. To know our self, or place, or community connections is an important step in delivering homes for us all.

8 Going home
Conclusions

Introduction

Home goes beyond bricks and mortar – it is feeling, family, roots, history, culture, stage, screen, shelter, self, freedom and trap. It may be a momentary feeling of community or a physical protective structure. Home is not always a taken-for-granted 'complacent' thing, as King (2017) suggests in an ideal world it would be. This is because of the potential for conflict and social depletion within the home relating to the duty and chores for one's own family. There can also be threats to home and precariousness of home in the private rented sector where tenancies are insecure; or indeed inability to physically access a place to live – homelessness. But home, when one feels 'at home' is a place of love and nourishment, a platform or stage which we can be complacent in knowing is there – a place from which we can perform our lives.

Whilst for many, home is a private thing – there is a space for wider community involvement in home-making. The duality of home – love and duty – and the messiness of meanings around housing as home, the intersections between place and identity, creates a complex picture which is evident throughout the book. If home is love, then it cannot be mandated by government or provided by builders. But government and builders can construct the dwellings, varied enough in design to meet a range of physical and cultural needs, where we as individuals – with the support of community, the safety-net of government welfare – can create home.

There is a need for support from government and society in creating and maintaining home. It is too important and precious to leave to the market alone to ensure sufficient physical places in which to create home. Adequate and safe housing, in which we can make homes, should be seen through a human rights lens. Constructing housing, regulating landlords in the private sector to ensure accommodation is safe and affordable should be a government priority. Government cannot build 'homes', but it can provide the financial and regulatory support to create the conditions necessary (security/affordability) for people to create their own home.

Conditions to create 'home'

Provision of housing is a very important part of creating and supporting 'home'. But it is not all. There are certain conditions, in addition to the box of bricks, which help housing to become home:

- *Security* that it is mine for as long as I need or want it – that I can leave it for a while and know it is mine to come back to, the tenancy secure, the land not bunded while I'm away.
- *Safety* of the physical dwelling, that it is not injurious to mine or my family's physical health; and that I am safe, from others, within the place.
- *Quality of space*, appropriate location of home, near to facilities, connected to nature and humanity, on a bus route to the swimming pool, the library – the leisure activities that enrich our lives.
- *Privacy* of place for my personal space, but with porous boundaries when I need to the home to breathe and to allow for:
- *Connectedness* within the walls and outside – with humans in the neighbourhood and far beyond, allowing for online worlds to support global connections, but not undermining the human connection within home.
- *Affordability* so that I can pay for home, without having to juggle three precarious jobs, be at threat of eviction, be ripped off. What is wrong with 'social' housing – what is its opposite? 'anti-social housing'? Creation and support of home is a social process; we forget this at our peril.

Conditions to support 'home'

There are a number of necessary conditions that should be in place to help support the creation of 'homes'. Government and civic society have a role to play in enhancing the position of these conditions.

Strong leadership in planning for home

Planning for, and living in, homes, is an emotional process. Chapter 2 discussed the emotionomics of home in the planning environment, and the need for negotiation. Government policy and local authority practice on the supply and delivery of 'homes' (housing) should better recognise this. Conflict (and the need for negotiation) should be recognised in the process of planning for homes. The antagonistic practices of place and identity connecting result, in some cases, of local communities saying no to new homes.

Local politicians' debate in this arena does not always show progressive leadership. MPs and councillors should recognise their duty to *all* their constituents, present and future, inter-generational, multi-racial – and demonstrate moral leadership in local planning debates.

Regulation of housing security and quality

Two of the conditions to create home (security and quality) need supporting through regulation of our increasingly privatised housing market. Quality of physical accommodation needs regulating for indicators of quality such as space standards, physical structure, value for money, proximity to services, equality of access to and treatment in the property across diverse groups.

Recognising the duality of home

This book has attempted show the duality (love and duty) of home – to throw the light and shade of home into a framework of planning and negotiation. Home is security and love, but is also conflict and control. It is a private space to be our authentic selves – a platform from which to perform. But it can also be a home-trap, a place of violence and fright, as we saw in Chapter 3. Sometimes home is a prison – a place where a partner controls, but it might also be a place where we gate ourselves in. Whilst the privacy afforded by home is what can make us feel safe, there is a space for government to ensure sufficient legal redress for women beaten in their houses, trapped in their place by a violent partner. Too many women and children have been killed in their domestic surroundings to continue using privacy as an excuse for doing nothing. The social housing sector, working with organisations like DAHA, are highlighting the issue of domestic and family violence and are using their position as 'always there' services to recognise the symptoms and intervene for the sake of safety, when necessary.

As a society, we should recognise the need for porous walls in our homes – to let the light in when it is dark and lonely – and to recognise the benefits of community connection for all of our wellbeing. We need to understand and properly value the work it takes to create home – the labour of cleaning, cooking, child-rearing, which should not be presumed as unpaid women's work today.

Take a more cautious approach to 'home screen'

Social and online communities can connect virtually, and appease isolation for those physically unable to get out and about. But they should be an addition to human connection, physical places – real-world experiences, not a replacement. I outlined in Chapter 4 how our homes – our walls – can physically screen us from the outside world. Our home screen on our computers and phones can also screen our identity by projecting an inauthentic performance of ourselves, our homes. Home already has a complicated intersection with place and identity – when we look at this through a lens of virtual online worlds, the notion of who we are and where we are present in place, becomes even more complex. The darker side of online worlds – exploitation and bullying – can invade our homes and put young people at risk. We see increasing evidence of the harmful effects of screen addiction and we should proceed with caution. Online connections can be beneficial for people who feel isolated – but there should be ways to design in human connection too – open doors and porous walls to allow people in, to help us feel at home.

Housing with support is the way to end homelessness

Housing and social policy is vital to a long term strategic approach to homelessness in its broadest sense. We also need a rapid response and a 'housing first' type of method to *ending street homeless*. Rather than leaving it to the market which has failed us and resulted in unacceptable rises in homelessness, we should see governments lead us in community approaches to halting the need for people to sleep on the street or sofa-surfing and other hidden homelessness. Homeless people have multiple and complex needs and so just providing the house, without the support to make it home can result in a 'revolving door' of entrenched and long-term homelessness. It is love that makes a home, not just the physical dwelling. Many housing practitioners want to show that care, that emotional support, but as we saw earlier in the book there is a tussle in the public and social housing sector between head and heart. The constraints resulting from austerity measures means it is harder to provide the vital support needed to create and maintain home.

Design accommodating spaces

We must go beyond house as home in order to get a better understanding of the meanings of home and the intersection of place and identity. Moreover, we should also move past the ingrained notion of house as dwelling. There are many different dwelling types from tent to trailer, from igloo to tree-house. By restricting the public imaginary to a box made of bricks, we exclude all other dwelling types as 'other'. There is a diversity of housing types across the globe, but also a narrow prevailing view of what home looks like. The resultant 'othering' of homes that don't look like a box made of bricks, creates a marginalisation of the residents in those places and accommodation types. Architects can lead the way in innovative design, but as a society we need to be more receptive to different uses of space. Common land can be play-park and temporary home to trailers – if the space is designed well and residents supported to be open to meanwhile use and shared communities. Common land use requires shared understandings and co-owned rules of use – and where this breaks down then regulation and action is necessary. Open space and common use does not mean allowing lawless places. Where all residents are supported and reassured (and where infractions and unfair misuse are dealt with) this multiplicity of place use can work well. The defining concepts of understanding home – place and identity – are ever moving constructs. As Massey (2005) confides, place is messy, it needs negotiation. Our conflicting notions of identity and our links with geographical space create a need to constantly re-negotiate place – if we are all to find our 'home' in a connected way, rather than from behind gates.

Look after ourselves so we can look after each other

Understanding what we mean by 'authentic' within a framework of performance of home is challenging. And yet it continues to be important to examine the characteristics and conditions to create home – for us all. Chapter 1 recognised the intersection between place and identity, and Chapter 7 explored further how this might help us to perform our authentic selves by feeling 'at home' with ourselves. Comprehending our own relationship with home is more likely to lead to a better understanding of how home manifests elsewhere for other people. Knowing who we are is not necessarily selfish, it is worth continued exploration in an attempt to avoid social hypoxia – a shared delirium leading to inertia and continued inaction on delivering homes for us all.

Valuing home

The value of home goes way beyond the economic cost of building a house, or the increasing value of housing. Financial measurement of the value of housing would be an inadequate method, because it would miss the emotional connection between place and identity which makes it so important. And yet, the government it seems, does not value housing or home in any meaningful sense. It sees money spent on building social housing as a burden of debt, rather than an investment. This is peculiar, as through policies like Right to Buy, it recommends personal financial investment in the property, without recognising the loss in wider social value. This policy results in absurdities such as councils renting back Right to Buy properties to house those in need, at a vastly inflated market rate. Councils pay housing benefit so that people can live in former Right to Buy properties now being let at rocket-high rents. Money is spent each month to pay rents, but it is not spent on longer term investment in building more social and affordable housing.

In his discussion on creating value for business, Mahajan (2016, pg 121) adapts a hierarchy of needs type of approach reaching a pinnacle where employees are inspired through a transformed understanding and a proximity to 'meaning' between their values and identity and the values of their organisation. I discussed this issue in the latter part of chapter seven on identity and authenticity – feeling at home at work. People who work in the social housing sector have been going through a phase of dissonance – a feeling that there may be a growing gap between the heart and the head of social housing provision. Value placed on 'surplus' (aka profit), and the ever increasing drive for elusive efficiencies, change the flavour of the sector. If value of home is put into better balance with the financial value of housing – those working on the frontline might start to feel more at home in their work again.

In our community-wide conversations, in political, media and social discourse, there is a need to re-establish our social and ethical values of home. Baker (2016) suggests we can address disconnected narratives by reconnecting ". . . *social policy to foundational values and beliefs within an emerging post neo-liberal consensus . . . with reference to social imaginary, spiritual capital and curating emerging spaces of ethical convergence and performative civil and political engagement*" (Baker, 2016, pg 259). Through a broad-based coalition of faith, political and other social actors – we need to all talk about the value of home.

On our way home

In understanding 'home', we should be better equipped to reframe housing politics, policy and practice for the future. If the duality – the light and shade – of home – of us, is recognised, then we can properly value home. We do need a longer-term political approach to the provision of housing for home – a clarity of social purpose and aim; moving beyond short-term priorities and 'business as usual' in the building and housing industry. Legislation and regulation around the building of houses, the negotiation of physical spaces, the connection of people and place can support what is both a private and public endeavour to make ourselves at home.

This short book has outlined the different ways we view home – and ourselves – in an effort to demonstrate the extraordinary value that housing can contribute to the making of home, and the vital importance of government and community in supporting home to happen. Whilst each one of us creates home for ourselves and our immediate family, wherever and whenever that may be; this must be in concert with our neighbours' needs. The diverse claims for home in the wider community must be negotiated and re-negotiated so we can all feel at home. There is a place for a more social approach to building housing as home, for governments to lead us in more proactive and progressive discursive spaces.

Home is located in the intersection between identity and place. Home allows us to perform our lives – in technical, empowering and creative ways. It can be a private, individual act to create home, but it does not happen in a vacuum. Billions of people across the planet are negotiating their journey to home, each with different ideas of place and identity, but sharing the same spaces and places. Home sweet home.

Bibliography

Agius, C. and Keep, D. (Eds) (2018) *The Politics of Identity: Place, Space and Discourse*, Manchester: Manchester University Press

Al Ramiah, A. and Hewstone, M. (2013) 'Intergroup Contact as a Tool for Reducing, Resolving and Preventing Intergroup Conflict', *American Psychologist*, 68(7), pgs 527–542

Amore, K., Baker, M. and Howden-Chapman, P. (2011, December) 'The ETHOS Definition and Classification of Homelessness: An Analysis', *European Journal of Homelessness*, 5(2), pgs 19–37

Andreou, A. (2015) 'It Was Only When I Became Homeless that the City's Barbed Cruelty Became Clear', *The Guardian G2*, pgs 4–7

Atkinson, R. and Blandy, S. (2017) *Domestic Fortress: Fear and the New Homefront*, Manchester: Manchester University Press

Atkinson, R. and Jacobs, K. (2016) *House, Home and Society*, London: Palgrave Macmillan

Bachelard, G. (2014) *The Poetics of Space*, London: Penguin Books Ltd (reprint of 1958 edition)

Baker, C. (2016) 'Faith in the Public Sphere – In Search of a Fair and Compassionate Society for the Twenty-first Century', *Journal of Beliefs & Values*, 37(3), pgs 259–272

Barry, J. and Porter, L. (2011) 'Indigenous Recognition in State-based Planning Systems: Understanding Textual Mediation in the Contact Zone', *Planning Theory*, 11(2), pgs 170–187

Baum, H. (2011) 'Planning and the Problem of Evil', *Planning Theory*, 10(2), pgs 103–123

Beadle, P. (2007) *Could Do Better!: Help Your Child Shine at School*, London: Doubleday

Beer, A. et al. (2016) 'Neoliberalism, Economic Restructuring and Policy Change: Precarious Housing and Precarious Employment in Australia', *Urban Studies*, 53(8), pgs 1542–1558

Berger, J. (1972) *Ways of Seeing*, London: Penguin Books Ltd

Bernheimer, L. (2017) *The Shaping of Us: How Everyday Spaces Structure Our Lives, Behaviour and Wellbeing*, London: Robinson (Kindle Edition)

Blunt, A. (2005) 'Cultural Geography: Cultural Geographies of Home', *Progress in Human Geography*, 29(4), pgs 505–515

Blunt, A. and Dowling, R. (2006) *Home*, Key Ideas in Geography, Hoboken: Taylor & Francis Ltd

Bordieu, P. (1991) *Language & Symbolic Power*, Cambridge: Polity Press

Bordieu, P. (1998) *Practical Reason*, Cambridge: Polity Press

Boughton, J. (2018) *Municipal Dreams: The Rise and Fall of Council Housing*, London: Verso

Breakwell, G. (2014) 'Identity and Social Representations', in Jaspal, R. and Breakwell, G. (Eds) *Identity Process Theory: Identity, Social Action and Social Change*, Cambridge: Cambridge University Press, pgs 118–134

Brewer, M. and Hewstone, M. (Eds) (2004) *Self and Social Identity*, Oxford: Blackwell Publishing

Brown, B. (2010) *The Gifts of Imperfection, Let Go of Who You Think You're Supposed to Be and Embrace Who You Are*, Center City: Hazleden

Buck, S. (1998) *The Global Commons: An Introduction*, Washington, DC: Island Press

Butler, J. (1999) *Gender Trouble: Feminism and the Subversion of Identity*, Second Edition, London: Routledge

Cairns, G., Artopoulos, G. and Day, K. (Eds) (2017) *From Conflict to Inclusion in Housing: Interaction of Communities, Residents and Activists*, London: UCL Press

Chapman, T. (1999) 'Houses of Doom' in Chapman T and Hockey J (1999), *Ideal Homes? Social Change and Domestic Life*, London, Routledge (pgs 147–160)

Chapman, T. and Hockey, J. (1999) *Ideal Homes? Social Change and Domestic Life*, London: Routledge

Chatwin, B. (1998) *The Songlines*, London: Vintage Penguin Random House

Clapham, D. (2002) 'Housing Pathways: A Post Modern Analytical Framework', *Housing, Theory and Society*, 19(2), pgs 57–68

Coleman, A. (1990) *Utopia on Trial: Vision and Reality in Planned Housing*, London: Hilary Shipman Ltd

Cosslett, R. (2015, 27th January) 'The Triumph of the Hive Mind: Why Is Gentrified London So Sterile and Dull?', *The New Statesman*, www.newstatesman.com

Crenshaw, K. (1991) 'Mapping the Margins: Intersectionality, Identity Politics, and Violence Against Women of Color', *Stanford Law Review*, 43(6), pgs 1241–1299

Darke, J. (1994) 'Women and the Meaning of Home', in Gilroy, R. and Woods, R. (Eds) *Housing Women*, London: Routledge, pgs 11–30

Davidson, J., Bondi, L. and Smith, M. (Eds) (2005) *Emotional Geographies*, London: Ashgate

De Certau, M. (1988) *The Practice of Everyday Life*, Berkeley: University of California Press

Dee, T. (Ed) (2018) *Ground Work: Writings on Places and People*, London: Jonathan Cape

Ders, H. (1990) *Community, Culture, Difference*, London: Lawrence and Wishart

Despres, C. (1991) 'The Meaning of Home: Literature Review and Directions for Future Research and Theoretical Development', *Journal of Architectural and Planning Research*, 8(2), pgs 96–114

Despres, C. and Lord, S. (2005) 'Growing Older in Postwar Suburbs: The Meanings and Experiences of Home', in Rowles, G. D. and Chaudhury, H. (Eds) *Home and Identity in Late Life*, New York: Springer, pgs 317–340

Doherty, J. and Edgar, B. (Eds) (2008) *In My Caravan, I Feel Like Superman*, St Andrews: Centre for Housing Research/FEANTSA

Donahue, E. (2010) *Room*, London: Little Brown

Dowling, R. and Power, E. (2012) 'Sizing Home, Doing Family in Sydney, Australia', *Housing Studies*, 27(5), pgs 605–619

Dryden, C. (1999) *Being Married, Doing Gender: A Critical Analysis of Gender Relationships in Marriage*, London: Routledge

Easthope, H. (2004) 'A Place Called Home', *Housing, Theory and Society*, 21(3), pgs 128–138

Elson, D. (2000) 'Progress of the World's Women 2000', *UNIFAM*, http://iknowpolitics.org/sites/default/files/progress_of_the_world_s_women_2000.pdf (accessed 15/4/18)

Emin, T. (1998) *My Bed Installation*, London: Tate Galleries

Fischer, F. and Gottweis, H. (Eds) (2012) *The Argumentative Turn Revisited: Public Policy as Communicative Practice*, London: Duke University Press

Fisher, R. and Ury, W. (1999) *Getting to Yes: Negotiating an Agreement Without Giving In*, London: Random House

Forester, J. (1999) *The Deliberative Practitioner: Encouraging Participatory Planning Processes*, Cambridge, MA: MIT Press

Forester, J. (2009) *Dealing With Differences: Dramas of Mediating Disputes*, Oxford: Oxford University Press

Foucault, M. (1967, March) 'Des Espace Autres', *Of Other Spaces: Utopias and Heterotopias*, Architecture/Mouvement/Continuité, October 1984 (Translated From the French by Jay Miskowiec)

Foucault, M. (1969) *The Birth of the Clinic: An Archaeology of Medical Perception*, Translated by A. Sheridan, London: Tavistock Publications

Foucault, M. (1977) *Discipline and Punish, the Birth of the Prison*, London: Penguin Books Ltd

Franklin, A. (2009, December) 'On Loneliness', *Geografiska Annaler: Series B, Human Geography*, 91(4), pgs 343–354

Gilman, C. (2018) *The Home: It's Work and Influence*, London: Create Space Independent (reprint of 1903 edition)

Gilroy, R. and Woods, R. (Eds) (1994) *Housing Women*, London: Routledge

Goffman, E. (1959) *The Presentation of Self in Everyday Life*, London: Penguin Books Ltd

Gold, T. (2017, 5th August) 'There Are Two Cornwalls: The Paradise of My Fantasies and the Place I've Moved To', *The Guardian Magazine*, pg 5

Goodhart, D. (2017) *The Road to Somewhere: The Populist Revolt and the Future of Politics*, London: Hurst & Company

Graham, S. (2011) *Cities Under Siege: The New Military Urbanism*, London: Verso

The Guardian (2017) 'One in Every 200 People in UK Are Homeless, According to Shelter', www.theguardian.com/society/2017/nov/08/one-in-every-200-people-in-uk-are-homeless-according-to-shelter (accessed 10/11/17)

Gunder, M. (2011) 'A Metapsychological Exploration of the Role of Popular Media in Engineering Public Belief on Planning Issues', *Planning Theory*, 10(4), pgs 325–343

Gurney, C. (1990) 'The Meaning of Home in the Decade of Owner Occupation', *Working Paper 88*, Bristol School for Advanced Urban Studies, University of Bristol

Harrison, T. (2018, 15th January) 'Alone Together: Who's Lonely and How Do We Measure It?', *RSA*, www.thersa.org (accessed 20/4/18)

Harvey, D. (2013) *Rebel Cities: From the Right to the City to the Urban Revolution*, London: Verso

Healey, P. (2006) *Collaborative Planning: Shaping Places in Fragmented Societies*, Second Edition, Basingstoke: Palgrave Macmillan

Healey, P. (2012) 'Performing Place Governance Collaboratively: Planning as a Communicative Process', in Fischer, F. and Gottweis, H. (Eds) *The Argumentative Turn Revisited: Public Policy as Communicative Practice*, London: Duke University Press

Heidegger, M. (1993) *Basic Writings*, San Francisco: Harper

Higson, A. (1984, July–October) 'Space, Place, Spectacle', *Screen*, 25, pgs 2–21

Hill, D. (2008) *Emotionomics: Leveraging Emotions for Business Success*, London: Kogan Page

Hockey, J. (1999) 'Houses of Doom', in Chapman, T. and Hockey, J. (Eds) *Ideal Homes? Social Change and Domestic Life*, London: Routledge, pgs 147–160

hooks, b. (1987) *Ain't I a Woman: Black Women and Feminism*, London: Pluto Press

hooks, b. (1994) *Outlaw Culture: Resisting Representations*, London: Routledge

Hudson, J. and Lowe, S. (2009) *Understanding the Policy Process: Analysing Welfare Policy and Practice*, Second Edition, Bristol: Policy Press

Innes, J. and Booher, D. (2010) *Planning With Complexity: An Introduction to Collaborative Rationality for Public Policy*, London: Routledge

Jacobs, J. (1961) *The Death and Life of Great American Cities*, New York: Modern Library (reprinted in 2011 for the 50th anniversary edition)

Jaspal, R. and Breakwell, G. (Eds) (2014) *Identity Process Theory: Identity, Social Action and Social Change*, Cambridge: Cambridge University Press

Jenkins, R. (2008) *Social Identity*, Third Edition, Abingdon: Routledge

Kabachnik, P. (2010a) 'Place Invaders: Constructing the Nomadic Threat in England', *Geographical Review*, 100(1), pgs 90–108

Kabachnik, P. (2010b) 'England or Uruguay? The Persistence of Place and the Myth of the Placeless Gypsy', *Area*, 42(2), pgs 198–207

Kaufman, S. and Smith, J. (1999) 'Framing and Reframing in Land Use Change Conflicts', *Journal of Architectural and Planning Research*, 16(2), pgs 164–180

Kemeny, J. (1995) *From Public Housing to the Social Market: Rental Policy Strategies in Comparative Perspective*, London: Routledge

Kemeny, J. (2005) *From Public Housing to the Social Market*, London: Routledge

Kemsley, R. and Platt, C. (2012) *Dwelling With Architecture*, London: Routledge

King, P. (2004) *Private Dwelling: Contemplating the Use of Housing*, London: Routledge

King, P. (2005) *The Common Place: The Ordinary Experience of Housing*, Aldershot: Ashgate

King, P. (2010) *Housing Boom and Bust: Owner Occupation, Government Regulation and the Credit Crunch*, London: Routledge

King, P. (2017) *Thinking on Home*, Abingdon: Routledge

Laclau, E. and Mouffe, C. (2001) *Hegemony and the Socialist Strategy: Towards a Radical Democratic Politics*, Second Edition, London: Verso

Laing, O. (2017) *The Lonely City: Adventures in the art of being alone*, Edinburgh: Canongate

Laws, D. and Forester, J. (2015) *Conflict, Improvisation, Governance: Street Level Practices for Urban Democracy*, London: Routledge

Lawson, J. (2006) *Critical Realism and Housing Research*, London: Routledge

Le Corbusier (1985) *Towards a New Architecture*, New York: Dover Publishing (reprint of 1927 edition)

Lefebvre, H. (1991) *The Production of Space*, Oxford: Blackwell Publishing

Le Grand, J. (2013) *Motivation, Agency, and Public Policy: Of Knights & Knaves, Pawns & Queens*, Paperback Edition, Oxford: Oxford University Press

Lenhard, J. F. (2018) *Making Better Lives – Home Making Among Homeless People in Paris*, Doctoral thesis, https://doi.org/10.17863/CAM.21752

Levitt, S. and Dubner, S. (2005) *Freakonomics: A Rogue Economist Explores the Hidden Side of Everything*, London: Allen Lane

Lindholm, C. (2008) *Culture and Authenticity*, Oxford: Blackwell Publishing

Lloyd, J. and Johnson, L. (2004) 'Dream Stuff: The Post-war Home and the Australian Housewife, 1940–60', *Environment and Planning D: Society and Space*, 22, pgs 251–272

Lord, S., Despres, C. and Ramadier, T. (2011) 'When Mobility Makes Sense: A Qualitative and Longitudinal Study of the Daily Mobility of the Elderly', *Journal of Environmental Psychology*, 31, pgs 52–61

Lukes, S. (1974) *Power: A Radical View*, Basingstoke: Macmillan Press Ltd

Madanipour, A. (2010) 'Connectivity and Contingency in Planning', *Planning Theory*, 9(4), pgs 351–368

Mahajan, G. (2016) *Value Creation: The Definitive Guide for Business Leaders*, London: Sage

Mahdawi, A. (2015, 15th January) 'Neighbourhood Rebranding: Wanna Meet in LoHo, CanDo or GoCaGa?', *The Guardian*, www.theguardian.com/cities

Mallett, S. (2004) 'Understanding Home: A Critical Review of the Literature', *Sociological Review*, 52(1), pgs 62–89

Maslow, A. H. (1943). 'A Theory of Human Motivation', *Psychological Review*, 50(4), pgs 370–396

Massey, D. (1994) *Space, Place and Gender*, Cambridge: Polity Press

Massey, D. (2005) *For Space*, London: Sage

McGarry, A. and Jasper, J. (Eds) (2015) *The Identity Dilemma: Social Movements and Collective Identity*, Philadelphia: Temple University Press

McKenzie, J. (2001) *Perform or else: from discipline to performance*, London: Routledge

McNaughton, C. (2008) *Transitions Through Homelessness: Lives on the Edge*, Basingstoke: Palgrave Macmillan

McVeigh, T. (2016, 11th December) 'Spikes, Railings and Water Are Weapons of "Dehumanising" Campaign Against Homeless', *The Observer*, pg 11

Meert, H., Stuyck, K., Cabrera, P., Dyb, E., Filipovic, M., Gyori, P., Hradecky, I., Loison, M. and Maas, R. (2008) 'The Changing Profiles of Homeless People: Conflict, Rooflessness and the Use of Public Space', in Doherty, J. and Edgar, B. (Eds) *In My Caravan, I Feel Like Superman*, St Andrews: Centre for Housing Research/FEANTSA, pgs 171–206

Menary, R. (Ed) (2010) *The Extended Mind*, Cambridge, MA: MIT Press

Millard, W. (2018) 'My Year With the Tribe', *BBC2 Documentary*, Episode One Aired Sunday 15th April

Minton, A. (2009) *Ground Control: Fear and Happiness in the Twenty-first Century City*, London: Penguin Books Ltd

Minton, A. (2017) *Big Capital: Who Is London For?* London: Penguin Books Ltd

Mintzberg, H. and Westley, F. (2001, Spring) 'Decision Making: It's Not What You Think', *MIT Sloan Management Review*, pgs 89–93

Modern Slavery Act (2015) Chapter 30, London: *The Stationery Office*. Online http://www.legislation.gov.uk/ukpga/2015/30/contents/enacted

Moore, J. (2000) 'Placing Home in Context', *Journal of Environmental Psychology*, 20, pgs 207–217

Moore and Coates v Secretary of State for Communities and Local Government & London Borough of Bromley and Dartford Borough Council and Equality and Human Rights Commission [2015] EWHC 44 (Admin)

National Audit Office (2017) *Homelessness*, London: NAO, pg 5, www.nao.org.uk/wp-content/uploads/2017/09/Homelessness.pdf

Nebehay, S. and Lewis, S. (2018, 7th March) '"Acts of Genocide" Suspected Against Rohingya in Myanmar – U.N.', *Reuters*, https://uk.reuters.com/article/uk-myanmar-rohingya-rights/acts-of-genocide-suspected-against-rohingya-in-myanmar-u-n-idUKKCN1GJ167

Nepo, M. (2018) *More Together than Alone: The Power of Community*, London: Rider Books

Newman, O. (1972) *Defensible Space: Crime Prevention Through Urban Design*, Basingstoke: Macmillan Press Ltd

Newton, J. (2014) *Parkland: When Caravan Is home*, Melbourne: Australian Scholarly

New York City (2015) *Mandatory Inclusionary Housing Policy*, www1.nyc.gov/assets/planning/download/pdf/plans-studies/mih/mih_report.pdf

Noor, P. (2018, 9th May) 'My Community Is Vehemently Against Travellers Settling on a Local Common. How Can I Challenge This?', *The Guardian*, www.theguardian.com/lifeandstyle/2018/may/09/tavellers-community-against-settling-local-common

O'Campo, P., Daoud, N., Hamilton-Wright, S. and Dunn, J. (2016) 'Conceptualizing Housing Instability: Experiences With Material and Psychological Instability Among Women Living With Partner Violence', *Housing Studies*, 31(1), pgs 1–19

Oliver, P. (2003) *Dwellings*, New York: Phaidon Press

Orlek, J. (2017) 'Sharing the Domestic Through Residential Performance', in Cairns, G., Artopoulos, G. and Day, K. (Eds) *From Conflict to Inclusion in Housing: Interaction of Communities, Residents and Activists*, London: UCL Press, pgs 180–198

Osman, O. and Busari, S. (2017, 27th June) 'Otodo Gbame: Landmark Ruling Gives Lifeline to Evicted Lagos Residents', *CNN*, https://edition.cnn.com/2017/06/27/africa/otodo-gbame-demolition/index.html

Ostrom, E. (1990) *Governing the Commons: The Evolution of Institutions for Collective Action*, New York: Cambridge University Press

Oyserman, D. (2004) 'Self-concept and Identity', in Brewer, M. and Hewstone, M. (Eds) *Self and Social Identity*, Oxford: Blackwell Publishing, pgs 5–24

Pain, R. (1991) 'Space, Sexual Violence and Social Control: Integrating Geographical and Feminist Analyses of Women's Fear of Crime', *Progress in Human Geography*, 15(4), pgs 415–431

Parsons, W. (1995) *Public Policy: An Introduction to the Theory and Practice of Policy Analysis*, Northampton: Edward Elgar Press

Petty, J. (2016) 'The London Spikes Controversy: Homelessness, Urban Securitisation and the Question of Hostile Architecture', *International Journal for Crime, Justice and Social Democracy*, 5(1), pgs 67–81. doi:10.5204/ijcsd.v5i1.286

Piazza, R. (2014) '. . . Might Go to Birmingham, Leeds . . . Up Round There, Manchester . . . and Then We Always Come Back Here . . .': The Conceptualisation of Place Among a Group of Irish Women Travellers', *Discourse & Society*, 25(2), pgs 263–282

Pile, S. and Keith, M. (Eds) (2004) *Place and the Politics of Identity*, London: Taylor & Francis Ltd

Podziba, S. (2012) *Civic Fusion: Mediating Polarized Public Disputes*, Chicago: American Bar Association

Porter, L. (2010) *Unlearning the Colonial Cultures of Planning*, Farnham: Ashgate

Porter, L. and Barry, J. (2015) 'Bounded Recognition: Urban Planning and the Textual Mediation of Indigenous Rights in Canada and Australia', *Critical Policy Studies*, 9(1), pgs 22–40

Price, S. and SanzSabido, R. (Eds) (2016) *Sites of Protest*, London: Roman & Littlefield

Putnam, R. (2010) *Bowling Alone: The Collapse and Revival of American Community*, New York: Simon & Schuster

Quicke, S. and Green, C. (2018, April) '"Mobile (Nomadic) Cultures" and the Politics of Mobility: Insights From Indigenous Australia', *Transactions*, Online first, https://doi.org/10.1111/tran.12243

Rai, S., Hoskyns, C. and Thomas, D. (2013) 'Depletion: The Cost of Social Reproduction', *International Feminist Journal of Politics*, pgs 86–105. doi:10.1080/14616742.2013.789641

Ravetz, A. and Turkington, R. (2011) *The Place of Home: English Domestic Environments, 1914–2000*, Abingdon: Taylor & Francis Ltd

Resolution Foundation (2018) *A New Generational Contract – The Final Report of the Intergenerational Commission*, Resolution Foundation, www.intergencommission.org

Reynolds, M. (1962) *Little Boxes*, Song (Covered by Pete Seeger in 1963)

Richardson, J. (2006) *The Gypsy Debate: Can Discourse Control?* Exeter: Imprint Academic

Richardson, J. (2007) *Providing Gypsy/Traveller Sites: Contentious Spaces*, York: Joseph Rowntree Foundation

Richardson, J. (Ed). (2010) *Housing and the Customer: understanding needs and delivering services*, Coventry: Chartered Institute of Housing

Richardson, J. (2011) *The Impact of Planning Circular 1/06 on Gypsies and Travellers in England*, Leicester: De Montfort University

Richardson, J. (2014) 'Roma in the News: An Examination of Media and Political Discourse and What Needs to Change', *People, Place and Policy Online*, 8(1), pgs 51–64

Richardson, J. (2016) 'Gypsy and Traveller Sites: Performance of Conflict and Protest', in Price, S. and SanzSabido, R. (Eds) *Sites of Protest*, London: Roman & Littlefield, pgs 179–194

Richardson, J and Codona, J. (2016) *Providing Gypsy and Traveller Sites: negotiating conflict*, York JRF/ Coventry CIH

Richardson, J (2016a) Unpublished survey responses for 'Resilience on the frontline', unpublished.

Richardson, J. (2017a) 'Precarious Living in Liminal Spaces: Neglect of the Gypsy-Traveller Site', *Global Discourse*, 7(4), pgs 496–515

Richardson, J. (2017b) 'Conflict Sites in a Time of Crisis: Negotiating a Space and Place for Gypsies and Travellers', in Cairns, G., Artopoulos, G. and Day, K. (Eds) *From Conflict to Inclusion in Housing: Interaction of Communities, Residents and Activists*, London: UCL Press, pgs 40–55

Richardson, J., Barker, L., Furness, J. and Simpson, M. (2014) *Frontline Futures: New Era, Changing Role for Housing Officers*, Coventry: CIH

Richardson, J. and O'Neill, R. (2012) 'Stamp on the Camps: The Social Construction of Gypsies and Travellers in Media and Political Debate', in Richardson, J. and Ryder, A. (Eds) *Gypsies and Travellers: Empowerment and Inclusion in British Society*, Bristol: Policy Press, pgs 169–186

Richardson, J. and Ryder, A. (Eds) (2012) *Gypsies and Travellers: Empowerment and Inclusion in British Society*, Bristol: Policy Press

Rousseau, J. (1998) *The Social Contract*, London: Wordsworth Editions (Originally published 1762)

Rowling, J. K. (1998) *Harry Potter and the Chamber of Secrets*, London: Bloomsbury

Roy, N., Dubé, R., Després, C., Freitas, A. and Légaré, F. (2018) 'Choosing Between Staying at Home or Moving: A Systematic Review of Factors Influencing Housing Decisions Among Frail Older Adults', *PLoS ONE*, 13(1)

Rutherford, J. (1990) 'The Third Space. Interview With Homi Bhabha', in Ders, H. (Ed) *Community, Culture, Difference*, London: Lawrence and Wishart, pgs 207–221

Sahlin, I. (2008) 'Urban Definitions of Places and People', in Doherty, J. and Edgar, B. (Eds) *In My Caravan, I Feel Like Superman*, St Andrews: Centre for Housing Research/FEANTSA, pgs 101–126

Salvation Army (2017) *Supporting Adult Victims of Modern Slavery: Update on the Sixth Year*, https://adobeindd.com/view/publications/97955a9d-1164-456e-a329-d14eadfc3ef6/7jz8/publication-web-resources/pdf/366_SA_Modern_Slavery_Report_2017_Digital3.pdf (accessed 15/4/18)

Sanyal, B. (2005) 'Planning as Anticipation of Resistance', *Planning Theory*, 4(3), pgs 225–245

Saunders, P. and Williams, P. (1988) 'The Constitution of the Home: Towards a Research Agenda', *Housing Studies*, 3(2), pgs 81–93

Sennett, R. (2018) *Building and Dwelling: Ethics for the City*, London: Penguin Books Ltd (Kindle Edition)

Shaw, J. and Shaw, H. (2015) 'The Politics and Poetics of Spaces and Places: Mapping the Multiple Geographies of Identity in a Cultural Post human Era', *Journal of Organisational Transformation & Social Change*, 12(3), pgs 234–256. doi:10.1080/14779633.2015.1101254

Shenai, S., Jury-Dada, S., McLeod, D. and Webb, M. (2018) *Safe at Home: The Case for a Response to Domestic Abuse By Housing Providers*, Gentoo Group, www.gentoogroup.com/media/1571446/2018-03-28-web-ready-safe-at-home-report.pdf

Shields, R. (1991) *Places on the Margin: Alternative Geographies of Modernity*, London: Routledge

Sigman, A. (2017) 'Screen Dependency Disorders: A New Challenge for Child Neurology', *Journal of the International Child Neurology Association*, http://jicna.org/index.php/journal/article/view/67

Silverman, C. (1982) 'Everyday Drama: Impression Management of Urban Gypsies', *Urban Anthropology*, v11 n3-4 pgs 377–98 Fall-Winter

Smith, Z. (2017) *Feel Free: Essays*, London: Penguin Books Ltd

Somerville, P. (1989) 'Home Sweet Home: A Critical Comment on Saunders and Williams', *Housing Studies*, 3(2), pgs 81–93

Somerville, P. (1997) 'The Social Construction of Home', *Journal of Architectural and Planning Research*, 14(3), pgs 226–245

Spinney, A. (2012) 'Home and Safe? Policy and Practice Innovations to Prevent women and Children Who Have Experienced Domestic and Family Violence From Becoming Homeless', *AHURI Final Report No.196*, Australian Housing and Urban Research Institute, Melbourne, www.ahuri.edu.au/publications/p50602/

Steiner, H. and Veel, K. (2017) 'Negotiating the Boundaries of Home: The Making and Breaking of Lived and Imagined Walls', *Home Cultures*, 14(1), pgs 1–5

Steward, B. (2000, March) 'Living Space: The Changing Meaning of Home', *British Journal of Occupational Therapy*, 63(3), pgs 105–110. doi:10.1177/030802260006300303

Sullivan, C. and Olsen, L. (2016) 'Common Ground, Complementary Approaches: Adapting the Housing First Model for Domestic Violence Survivors', *Housing and Society*, 43(3), pgs 182–194

Susskind, L. (1996) *Dealing With an Angry Public: The Mutual Gains Approach to Resolving Disputes*, New York: The Free Press

Tajfel, H. (1981) *Human Groups and Social Categories: Studies in Social Psychology*, Cambridge: Cambridge University Press

The Traveller Movement and Others – v – J D Wetherspoon Plc, Central London County Court, 18 May 2015, HHJ Hand QC

Townsend, M. (2016, 14th February) 'Top Author Joins "Mass Trespass" Over Privatising Public Spaces', *The Guardian*, pg 6

Tuan, Y. (1977) *Space and Place: The Perspective of Experience*, Minneapolis: University of Minnesota Press

Turkle, S. (2011) *Alone Together: Why We Expect More From Technology and Less From Each Other*, New York: Basic Books

Tyler, A. (1992) *Dinner at the Homesick Restaurant*, London: Vintage Penguin Random House

Vasudevan, A. (2017) *The Autonomous City: A History of Urban Squatting*, London: Verso

Visoka, G. (2018) 'Agents of Peace: Place, Identity and Peacebuilding', in Agius, C. and Keep, D. (Eds) *The Politics of Identity: Place, Space and Discourse*, Manchester: Manchester University Press, pgs 71–87

Walby, S., Towers, J., Balderston, S., Corradi, C., Francis, B., Heiskanen, M., Helweg-Larsen, K., Mergaert, L., Olive, P., Palmer, E., Stöckl, H. and Strid, S. (2017) *The Concept and Measurement of Violence against Women and Men*, Bristol: Policy Press

Warrington, M. (2001) '"I Must Get Out": The Geographies of Domestic Violence', *Transactions of the Institute of British Geographers*, 26(3), pgs 365–382

Weedon, C. (2004) *Identity and Culture: Narratives of Difference and Belonging*, Maidenhead: Open University Press

Whitworth, D. (2018, 24th May) 'Sextortion: Big Rise in Victims With Tens of Thousands at Risk', *BBC*, www.bbc.co.uk/news/newsbeat-43433015

Wilson, J. and Kelling, G. (1982, March) 'Broken Windows', *Atlantic Monthly*, 249(3), pgs 29–38

Wolfe, T. (1982) *From Bauhaus to Our House*, London: Cardinal

Index

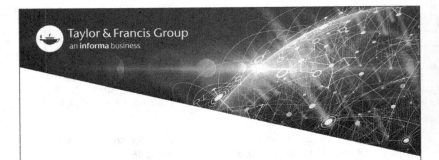